I0402289

Born Rich of Two Souls

When Some Say I Have Not One

Author: Sue Blondin

ISBN: 9781797937366
Imprint: Independently published

TABLE OF CONTENTS

I have started this montage of my thoughts and life so many times and so many times as, people often do, I have given up, forgotten about, found something more entertaining or been intimated by the final product. So here it is, attempt between 17 to 476 thousand some-odd. My name is Sue and I was diagnosed with both Borderline Personality Disorder and Bipolar I (one) mixed some 476 thousand attempts ago. As you will learn I was an ideally lucky case of early onset Bipolar so my parents' inept ability to handle it led me to also develop a personality disorder. This very occurrence is the reason for the title, the aforementioned montage of a mentally ill woman's ramblings. I was born rich of two souls when some say I have not one.

Some of the things you see written here are very personal and very deep. I don't expect that there will be no one to laugh at my pain but I'm hoping that if this could help one person struggling to find themselves or confused and detached from reality. Maybe the need to do everything on their own because they don't need anyone, then my effort was worth it. I'd like those individuals out there, the cutters and the self-medicated addicts or the scared and crying, stubborn ones to know they are not alone, and they don't have to be. Take it from the foremost expert on being strong and stubborn- help is better. Friends are better. Giving love and taking it just as strongly as you would your own self-punishment is better. I didn't always think so and I am in no way cured or better or happier. Letting my fiancé help me still pisses me off but he holds me and tells me how beautiful and strong I am and how I'm not broken but merely squeaky- that's better.

One of the things I am going to be sharing with you which is very personal to me, are tidbits of my "angry journal". An "angry journal" is the book I most write in when my emotions have become uncontrollable and they need to get out. Just air on the side of caution as some of that may contain triggers and the last thing, I find myself urging to do is trigger the people I'm trying to reach.

I won't be going into detail on the images you may see from my journal as they can speak for themselves but one thing to keep in mind when looking at them is every one of them was during some type of 'episodic behavior' or another. Although they may speak for themselves, their explanation is fuzzy.

Otherwise whatever you see may likely seem like unorganized rambling …. And it is… but to a borderline individual the contents and directions will make perfect sense. For those of you without a borderline affliction, try and see the directions of the contents as the way I see it. Read through the pages knowing that to me… it all makes sense. To me…. That's how my mind sees it.

On another note, the characters although real have had some liberties given to them including false names. You understand.

"

Little girl reflecting back

Both of us still broken

Scars faded yet still avail

Childhood tokens

Good then, same as good now

Neither one can reach

Lectures linger and carryon

But never did they teach

Are either of them even there?

"

THE MONSTERS STARTED FIRST

My mother taught me to see the good in everybody and everything. She taught me every day that life was meant for each and every one of us. She taught me that there were no bad people- only bad actions. Sometimes I would dream that the world would be filled with rainbows and the people that were sad or angry- and those that had done bad things- could be taken across this rainbow and made different. I would wish they were brought happiness in a way that would make them see the world a bit brighter and life a bit changed.

As much as I would love to say I stopped seeing that shortly after my fifth birthday, I cannot. You'll find later in this tiny bit of a chapter that as I got older those waiting for the rainbow standing atop something they've destroyed became in some way, a relationship for me. I never have stopped dreaming of rainbows.

The same mother that taught me to believe in rainbows also had signs of bipolar which, although never confirmed, was discussed at length and with great determination. This same mother- seemed to have spread it to me as I would find I had the lucky advantage of as I got older.

"Here dear, have the plaque that we discussed."

I was so young when the symptoms revealed themselves that I didn't know what was happening to me. I didn't know who I was, and sometimes didn't know where I was. When did the house change? When did everyone around me change? I would have outbursts that would hurt those around me that I loved. Unprovoked and confusing to everybody. My parents just assumed they were temper tantrums, some way to get what I want. They were too hard for me to explain so I would just let them carry on with what they believed happened.

It's as if I woke one morning in a different place and a different person all together. A wingless butterfly in a world of dragons. I remember the absolute fear that struck me down like a hot iron against my bare skin. Of course, I mustn't speak a word of it to anyone in my family because they would fear me mad. So, I endured the changes and the miseries in silence as my mind continued to break.

The monsters started first. Everywhere around me, surrounding me, I could see the fangs, and the wrath. The ugliest of them all were the teachers and others employed to care, and let's not forget the care takers that did too much teaching. I fail to remember telling anyone about the monsters but soon people started finding out The family, the neighbors, even the school administrators. My secret has been cast! I have been found out! And nobody could explain them, nobody would admit to seeing them. I knew differently and I had to keep myself safe. I'd let them all have their fairytale love affairs and all too fancy dinner parties. All the while mocking me and scowling from afar.

To make matters worse is the monsters gave way to other monsters just by association. I was raised that by nature, people are kind and the world is just, especially those we are made to respect like teachers, fireman, police officers, judges, military folks. How was the world so blind that most of these respected figures were not to be respected but feared? They had the power to tear you down. They had the power to hurt you.

There was one instance in first or second grade- god I am too old if I cannot remember single digits- when my teacher, called us all up to the front of the classroom for a relay race of sorts. The race intention, you ask? The intention of the whole hoopla was pointing out parts in a sentence. Simple. Sentence. Structure.

One of the girls in my class, fancy free with her blond little curls and her perfectly cute pink sneakers Now this girl, let me explain how perfect and lovable she was. This girl used to like to burn my hands with pens merely because I wouldn't flinch. You know how you run the pen fast across a surface and it makes the tip hot enough to burn? I was her own personal little freak. Well needless to say, I was going up against her in the sentence relay. With every ounce of my being I did not want her to win. I could feel it with every bit of me. This wasn't one of those "I have to make mommy and dad proud" moments. This was utter terror and anger, rolled up in one nice big package. Looking back now I still can't imagine any moment like that where I wasn't at the very least terrified. Most of the terrifying situations you hear about aren't some first or second grade relay race. To this day I don't know why I bundled it all up that day and bundled it so tight that I managed to just make myself more of a freak.

So, when our turn was up, I ran my little legs as fast as I could, in corrective shoes, to the front of the board- and panicked. Straight out panicked. Instead of writing something somewhat educated to the relay race topic at hand- if you don't recall- parts of a sentence. Instead of saying something as simple as "subject", I wrote noun. Noun! I was mortified. To make it worse my monster teacher turned to me and sent me to the principal's office because "I might be having one of those spells again."

It happened once in central school that I can remember. Once. Once where I could not control it and experienced, what I later found to be called, episodic behavior in class. Since then my teachers had decided that every little thing was an episode and they were not equipped to handle it. Next best thing, send me to the principal's office. So off I went. I proved nothing to Miss Blonde Curls Pink Shoes, or my teacher. I just came across as a mentally challenged freak who can't muster up something as simple as "subject".

In that scenario, the teacher, who should have been a mentor to me. Someone I could trust. Her and Miss Blonde Curls Pink Shoes teamed up that day. My imagination ran rampant and what I saw was them both leaned back in their chairs holding their jovial bellies firm as they laughed and laughed. I'm supposed to trust my teachers and at the very least the schoolmates. How could I possibly return here should they not trust and love me as I do them. I couldn't fear or hate. All I could muster was defeat. They had won.

Another instance, and probably one of the most damaging to me was around the same year, maybe a bit before. I frequented my mother's friend's house at the top of our street. I liked to play with their dog, and at the same time found myself oddly attached to my mother's friend's daughter named Hellen. Hellen was several years my senior and was one of the coolest kids in middle school. Almost high school!

I was there all the time as one of the group. They poked harmless fun at me, and they let me listen to music and sing along with them. Hellen was friends with some of the nicest and attractive guys (well boys), also my senior. Some of them smoked cigarettes and took pills from their parent's medicine cabinet. Each day I could spend there amongst the 'cool kids' was one less day that I would have been otherwise deemed 'not normal'. Always days filled with normalcy and smiles.

I was sorely mistaken. Monsters attacked one day. The fiercest I would probably ever see. Hellen and I were lounging on the bed listening to 'Poison' by Alice Cooper when some of her friends showed up, including her boyfriend Adam. Adam was the cutest, but the biggest of the monsters.

Adam brought Hellen's dog up to the room and as I started to get up, Adam stopped me but putting his hand against the back of my shoulder stating that it'll be easier for the dog from behind. Shaken, I immediately flipped around when he pushed me back over. By now, I was very frightened. The boys' eyes sank into their sockets with a reddish glow and their lips curled outwards as their teeth gave way to dripping fangs underneath. I remember starting to tear up and tremble a little, almost as if my body assumed, they would stop were they to see the fear growing in me.

I looked over at Hellen for help, but she had become demonic as well. She grew fangs and claws that dripped with blood. Her eyes became stained red starbursts. I may have been little, but I saw a horror movie or two that taught me bedrooms and boys that are mean, are not safe. The trembling got worse and I can still hear them talking about how nobody would believe me should I attempt to speak of this to anyone. They went on and on, with every second of growing misery, about how I was a little freak and that anyone would think I was making it up to get attention.

"Not the dog," I remember crying. "I won't do it." At this point I was back in a seated position screaming to Adam that they liked me and were supposed to be nice to me. "We are your friends Sue," he repeated trying to push me back onto the bed. "Just let him lick you," I screamed, "No" as many times and loud as I could. I didn't know fully what was happening but remember my face starting to warm up and my limbs growing weaker. Next thing I know, talons were released, and Adam kicked Selvie (the dog) clear across the face. Selvie let out a ghastly yelp and ran from the room and disappeared down the stairs. That moment, I remember screaming for the dog and smacking at Adam with no avail. It felt as if the blood started to drain from my body.

When Adam finally released his grasp, I mustered up the courage to get up and leave the room. I went downstairs and poked around in the living room trying to check on Selvie. I found her behind the arm chair and she immediately came to greet me. Thankfully she was okay. I don't think I was very much okay. These kids were supposed to be my friends. Hellen was the daughter of my mom's best friend. I should've been safe in that house, but I wasn't.

To this day, I can feel the tension that invaded my body when they walked Selvie into the room and I can see the memory, clear as day, of Selvie being kicked. And that yelp. No one could forget that yelp. Those monsters have haunted me to this very day.

But I digress, moving on to the subject at hand, My younger life, the people around me, the monsters. "It wouldn't affect me," I told myself, swore to myself. Oh, but it did affect me. Greatly affected me to be more precise. These monsters were talking about me, judging me, even when I had done absolutely nothing to warrant such verdicts. I was behaving the way little girls were supposed to. I ate my vegetables and said "please" and "thank you". If I was doing everything 'right' how were they judging me? What were they seeing that was so 'off' – so not normal?

Almost thirty years later and I still don't know what they see. I still can't figure out what it is I am doing that's not 'just like them'. I used to blame the scars but they can't always see them so it can't be that. Can people see the scars behind the fabric? Is it a sense they have?

It's important to realize however that not everyone was a monster and although they never fully became extinct, they became less and less prevalent as years went on. Now, many of them become monsters just some of the time. Just glimpses here and there, always in those you trusted the most. Take my mother- or momma as she was to me.

Momma was an amazing woman, the most beloved and fierce woman I had ever met. There was a power to her, whether super or magical, it was a power to be reckoned with. In fact, she was a woman to be reckoned with. Momma most likely had bipolar, as I found out later in life, so when she was on point, she was on, but when she was off… she grew fangs larger than most.

There are too many stories to write about my mother but I'll let you in on a little glimpse of how she was. It started when I was far too little notice. The bad days. The drinking. The manipulation.

When I had first started hurting myself momma would do one of two things. She'd put on a real nice show for my father about how I did it to hurt her and would carry-on as if she was the victim or she would just ignore it all together as if I wasn't screaming for help and understanding.

When I would accidentally break something momma would always- always- accept my apology and forgive the accident but then when she switched either that day or days down the road I would no longer be forgiven and she would punish me.

When my sister was 17 there was an argument over a sweater that momma insisted was hers, but it was not. Momma insisted she stole it. This one, stupid argument, cost my sister her home.

There was one day where momma had gone from her sweet loving self to a fierce monster in the blink of an eye. I was living in my first apartment in Nashua when momma called one Saturday morning at about seven o'clock. I didn't get to the phone because I was pouring myself a cup of coffee but figured instead of calling her back right away only to let her go in a few minutes, I would wait until after my coffee and shower to give her a call back. Well, sweet and innocent momma suddenly started calling my phone every minute and each voicemail was worse than the last. The messages graduated from "Suzie, it's momma. Call me back" to "Susan! This is your mother! You better call me back right away!" in a matter of about ten minutes. Momma grew fangs quick. There was many a similar voicemail or incident with her until I just couldn't take it anymore. At this point, I had no idea she was truly sick- it was just an idea. I thought the proof is in the pudding and maybe momma was just a bitch after all and all the kindness and don't judge mentality was just a façade.

I left my mother that year. I thought I was making the right choice. There was no way I could be the angel she described when she bore fangs so long and sharp. But as it turns out, I was my mother's angel. The one thing she hated to live without. Momma has since passed and I lost my opportunity to return to her open arms and tell her I'm sorry for leaving. I have lost the opportunity to tell her that she was sick and I forgive all the wicked moments. I pray to the gods every day that momma is finally at peace and that she knows I regret leaving her and will for the rest of my days.

So, we've talked about the all-time monsters and the occasional monsters, even the monsters you didn't see coming. The last and scariest of them all, the monster you never caught until it was too late. I have one of those whom I used to be unbelievably close to. We told each other everything and she was the woman I looked up to, given she was six years my senior and not sick in the head (I apologize, mentally ill). My sister. Where do I begin? I think my therapist put it best when she said that typically mentally-inept parents, i.e. sick mom and emotionally handicapped dad, will either bless the Earth with a narcissist or a borderline (or something similar with dysregulated emotions). Obviously, I am the latter, but my sister wasn't born mentally-healthy after all.

For those of you that don't know a narcissist is an individual with exaggerated self-importance, a need for admiration or adoration, and exploitative behavior. In short, they lack true empathy and they fool almost everyone around them. She had me fooled for 36 years. Basically, the empathy and emotion tub fell off the truck and ran me over and missed her! Don't get me wrong, she plays a good game. She makes people think she's charitable and loving but it's a ruse, it's what she's supposed to do so she does it but when she didn't like that she couldn't control me anymore- at 36- she just stopped calling. She stopped texting. She stopped including me in her life all-together, but she made sure to carry on about how horrible I was when it suited her (specifically to my dad and his wife). She's a monster to trump them all- and I still have her on speed dial.

The monsters were so hard and real for me because regardless of momma's occasional outbursts, I was raised to love everybody, everything and life itself. Because of the BPD I also learned to give trust where trust was not always reasonable. So, when that trust was broken, the culprits turned astray, and I was able to see them for who they truly were. Monsters. The pearly-whites gave way to dripping fangs and the colorful- once trustworthy- eyes became squinted and red. Their very souls would turn to ash and all the while. I was guilty and punishable for letting their made-up masquerade play trickery on my very being. I was guilty for letting them into my heart, and my life.

I was guilty for letting the monsters in and I often wondered if my passionate trust is what caused them to change or if they were always just wolves in sheep's clothing. It was impossible to tell but either way, I was to blame. If they were always monsters, I was to blame for trusting and loving them. When I failed to see their true nature and later fear them when they bore their true form without disgust, I was to blame. I was to blame because they were due the level of trust I wielded until they became bored or too burdened that they grew fangs and dead eyes. Like previously mentioned, either scenario would have been my fault.

Never did I learn either. In relationships I was misguided or pushed, in familial relationships I couldn't fully hide my true nature before they grew too tired of me too soon. I was the forgotten email about the grandparent's anniversary, the forgotten phone call about Christmas dinner or the seating chart that had just too little room. Because of how I was and how I acted, everyone grew tired and eventually everyone forgot. The classic coin in my family, "oh that's just Suzie being Suzie." So, it stands to reason that if the family coins such a term and believes it without reserve and I have the utmost trust in them and their opinions, it must be true.

"

Teeth that gnash

The blessed pain

Take pieces and pieces

Won't you

Show me those claws

So I may display the parts to tear

I am sorry you are what you are

Because I am what I am

"

I CAN DO IT MYSELF

Early in life, very early in fact, I learned how to take care of myself. I learned so strongly to fend for myself that It became who I was, an innate part of me that would never chip away. You see, momma was sick, and dad worked all the time. But when dad was home and saw this trait in me, he would become confused and question what kind of child I was. He would fight with my mother, "it's not normal, you raised her wrong." The problem with that statement I so often heard was nobody raised me. That was most of the problem wasn't it? Later in life I would find out was 'borderline personality disorder with avoidant traits. Avoidant traits.

Attachment theory describes bonds and relationships formed with others. The effects of these relationships and bonds on a maturing individual will influence our attachment style. Basically, how we experience closeness with others.

Avoidant attachment occurs with an emotionally absent or abusive caregiver/parent. An invalidating environment. To avoid feelings of rejection the child will become self-reliant and independent. They learn to stay silent on any issue that they may be dealing with rather than seeking help.

I saw a comic once that portrayed that diagnosis perfectly. It was only about three or four frames but in frame one you saw a woman standing by the door and a baby playing with a set of blocks. In the next frame you saw the woman, assuming the baby's mother, holding her throat and laying on the ground. In the same frame you see the baby in the same posture as before paying no mind to the mother on the ground. The third frame shows the mother being taken in a stretcher all the while the baby was in the same posture. The last frame shows the baby by himself, In the same posture, playing with his blocks. The baby showed no need or worry about the mother being gone. He didn't need anyone. They would have just rejected him anyway.

I'm sure many of you reading this with a similar diagnosis remembers growing up watching all the other children being cared for when they were sick or hurt and thinking to yourself "what is their issue?" I would often find myself in repetition with the statement "I can do it myself" or the ever-popular term "I'm fine". But we were never fine, were we? Even though we seemed strong because we could do it all with little to no guidance or we could take care of ourselves when we were hurt or ill. We were never fine. We had voices screaming to us "don't be a burden do it yourself". We were never fine; we should not have developed this avoidant personality. We should have been kids who get ice cream when they skin their knee or tucked in when they were sick.

It started gradually for me from the flu when I didn't want to wake my parents, as I was practically crawling on the bathroom floor, or the twisted ankle I had to try and walk normal on when anyone was around. Even the times I would cut or burn myself and had to crawl above the linens to get the bandages. I remember having to hold one end of the gauze with my thumb bent in an awkward position to wrap around my own arm when I could barely reach the mirror. Dad would be shocked days later when he saw the freshly healed wound. Momma wasn't surprised though. She would confront dad about how a child should not hide such things and my dad again would tell her she was raising me wrong.

Raising me wrong? I'm screaming for help for someone to yell and tell me that cutting myself is wrong. Burning myself. Is. Wrong. Nobody ever did yell that at me, instead they would question why I couldn't be like the other kids. That was all. If the normal kids lived like I did and hurt themselves and everyone around them. If normal kids got dogs kicked in their faces and was taught how to dry-hump alongside their freak neighbor before third-grade. If normal kids saw any of it, they would fail too. I was quick to learn that I was a burden, or I wasn't good enough, or I was 'just wrong'.

When I was 11 years old, I had major surgery on my foot. I was born so pigeon toed that I could hardly walk and even though they fixed much of the problem with bandages and braces and corrective shoes, they couldn't fix the last bit until I stopped growing. Anyway, I digress. When I was 11, I had major surgery that would cost me four nights and five days in the hospital. Parkland Medical to be exact. During this time my dad was responsible for driving me because momma had just gotten new teeth and they didn't fit right so she wouldn't be seen in public. It was one of momma's bad weeks. So, dad brought me to the hospital which was a good start but when he got there, he told me he was going to wait in the waiting room and will come visit me when they get me into a room after surgery. I went through pre-op and then about an hour later moved into surgery, alone. When I woke up from the surgery, I was in my hospital room- not in the pediatric ward as expected- and as promised dad was there waiting. I remember he didn't say much until he started pushing the nurses' button frantically because I was terribly sick from the morphine, they had me on- which I was allergic to. Dad forgot that.

Anyway, the entire time dad spent in that hospital room with me I could visibly see the discomfort on his face. He wanted no more to be there than I wanted to have just had that horrific surgery. I kept telling him that he was free to go and that I was fine, but I could tell that he knew the right thing to do was to stay there, at least until I was able to fall back asleep. But I didn't want to be the 'right thing to do'. If he didn't want to be there as a father than I didn't want him there. Eventually dad left and I would see him once more before they picked me up five days later to bring me home.

The first two days in the hospital I couldn't eat anything because dad forgot to write on the form that I was a vegetarian and the hospital cafeteria kept sending me up food like turkey and ham. One time it was meatloaf if I remember correctly. It was not until one of the nurses questioned me on it did, they realize I didn't eat meat. She had the cafeteria immediately send me up some vegetable soup and toast. I was so embarrassed. Not because dad didn't care enough to tell them, but the gentleman bringing up the food took a special trip. But I was so grateful because I was so hungry. I can remember leveling that toast and the nurse looked at me as one of those starving kids I would see on TV. I figure dad's oversight on the whole 'vegetarian thing' must have been a hurried attempt to fill out the paperwork because there was too much to do - it was just a memory lapse.

Through all this, I remember the nurses scurrying about, glancing into my room as I lay there doing my logic puzzles. They all looked at me with a sense of concern and seeming disgust. I remember thinking to myself that I must have done something to offend one of them and all the others were following suit in their distaste for me. "But what did I do?" I thought to myself. Not until later in life did I learn that they were not spiteful towards me but were in fact worried that I was a child, not in the pediatric ward, by myself for so long- with no family around. No family there that could tell them I was allergic to morphine or that I was a vegetarian. No family there to tell them that I would not want to offend anybody by pushing the nurse's button when I was sick or asking the sandwich guy to remove the meat off the sandwich. That wasn't the right thing to do- asking those things of the nurses would be offensive. I felt shamefaced that the nurses scurried around worried about me when they didn't have to. I was fine. Which leads to me to another time.

Some smaller scale situations range from the beehive that overtook my clubhouse. When I was younger my father refused to let me have a treehouse no matter how much I begged. For I am not coordinated you see and it would have ended quite badly. Instead my father made me this grand clubhouse- up to code even. It had two floors with windows and a set of safely high monkey bars. It had a little round door with stairs that led up to it. The clubhouse was just fantastic, the best place to be. Well, one year a bee had built a nest in the dome ceiling atop the second story. I couldn't possibly go in it now. So for weeks my dad kept asking me why I wasn't using the clubhouse and I kept making excuse after excuse until finally one day I just said "I don't want the stupid clubhouse anymore." But I did want the clubhouse and if I had been able to recognize the heartache on my father's face back then as complete sadness maybe I would have been smart enough to just ask him to get rid of the beehive. But I didn't recognize the look. I didn't recognize that because I was too stubborn and proud to ask for help that I had hurt my father. So think of that when you don't realize that your avoidant personality hurts more than yourself.

So there were times like the hospital where my dad didn't come across as so great and then there were times like the beehive where I didn't come across as so great.

Point in fact, my father is an amazing man. He never beat me or starved me. He never locked me in a room without light or a bathroom. He did none of those things. The only things dad was guilty of was being neglectful (to a point) and giving up. When he found out I was sick, I was very little, and he did not believe it. I couldn't possibly have a mood disorder- it was all just a phase. Just like the rest of my family, it was always just a phase.

The doctors would explain to my parents what was wrong, what was different I should say, with me. Because they had such little work being done with BPD at that age and I also had undiagnosed bipolar it was tough for my dad to recognize the words on the paper as his daughter. I should say, most likely, that regardless of what the 'papers' and 'pamphlets' told him he wouldn't have read them anyway. If I was sick, it looked bad on him, and he would not have that.

This avoidance has followed me my entire life. The always having to be right, and stronger than everyone mentality is a literal haunt upon my very core. It hasn't just stopped with 'I'm fine' and 'I can take care of myself' complexes either. The situation at hand, is I avoid familial structure and closeness in general.

At this very moment. I have my sister who I have not spoken to in months. That whole scenario started with her telling me my friends inject themselves into my life and she didn't like my fiancé or that I was so close to his family. I have my father who doesn't know what to expect from me and better yet doesn't even know how to talk to me. And momma's dead. She left me like I left her.

Then let's bring in my fiancé's family. All of them that I know are wonderful. Moms as I call her but can't possibly to her face- fault on my part- is much like my mother in a way. She has a big heart and she often gives advice, typically not followed but warranted all the same. Then there's his step dad who I find myself admiring quite often. He's strong and quiet, speaks up when he needs to. Then you have his brother and sister and all his nieces and nephews who are very kind and fancy-free. None of them- none- have judged the scars or talked down to me because I am sick. None of them have done any of the things my own family does.

Yet still, I don't embrace them. I just can't. I am hoping that one day before we are married, I can call moms, 'moms', to her face. I hope that one day I can embrace them for what they are. Nice people who welcomed me as one of their own. A family. Until that time, I have attempted to get better at going to the birthday parties or the barbeques, but mostly for my fiancé's sake. Not mine as It should be. I shouldn't need to become stressed or anxious for a family barbeque, especially with such kind and wonderful people. I shouldn't face any of that, but I do. I get anxious at the term family and grow slightly disoriented at the 'right thing to do.'. These people aren't 'the right thing to do' as I was taught. They are family and I should embrace it.

Once there was a little girl
Like any other little girl
Dad worked
And mommy enjoyed her quiet time
Such hope and such promise
Such a smart little girl
Such an energetic little girl
Such a happy little girl
But dad worked
And mommy enjoyed her quiet time
Little girls notice
Little girls can see
Dad's not there
And mommy is sick
Little girls are alone
But little girls are strong
Little girls are alone
But little girls are confused
Little girls wouldn't get any stronger
When little girls are alone
Little girls won't know care
And these little girls won't understand love
And these little girls will perish
And these little girls will be nothing

"

Little girls
Shouldnt hurt
Little girls
Shouldnt have to choose
Little girls
Shouldnt choose wrong and life
is over for good.

a There comes
a time in everyones life
Where they know death is coming

I came for me
but I didnt die
It comes again
and again & again
am I so bad that
it wont take me?

27

OH WHERE, OH WHERE MIGHT SUZIE BE?

The hiding, oh the hiding. For those of you with simiiar afflictions to an individual with Borderline Personality or Bi-Polar you know full-well what the term 'hiding' means. For those of you not 'in the know' as us lucky folks, hiding Is the term used to describe the "I am fine" scenario. We learn very quickly, the need to appear happy and normal. This hiding, or more clinically called "apparent competence" keeps us safe. Not safe in the term most commonly coined but safe from judgement, from having to explain ourselves. We need to appear normal and happy and normal and calm and **normal**.

As stated by Marsha Linehan, author of "Cognitive-Behavorial Treatment of Borderline Personality Disorder",

"Apparent competence refers to the tendency of borderline individuals to appear competent to cope with everyday life at some times, and at other times to behave (unexpectedly to the observer) as if the observed competencies did not exist"

When I was very young, the tempers and uncotrolled emotions started- until my parents walked in the room. Once there, I was the picture of the happy child they had hanging up on the wall. At that age, the hiding was more for lack of understanding what I was feeling- or even what was happening. So it became the safety net so often used against either having to come up with a viable reason for the outburst or stating that I didn't really know what the matter might have been. Also, the outbursts caused a feeling of great shame or later guilt so why make an already very uncomfortable situation worse. And if you recall normalcy and the strength to carry myself through life without help was also an integral part of my childhood.

Subsequently although I don't fully understand the need for this apparent conpentence myself- even today- those three things aforesaid would be enough cause. Normalcy, shame, and strength.

There were times, however, when I wasn't so strong and couldn't pretend to be so normal. It happened often when I was about five or six.

One particular incident when I was about five not only showed my Mr. Hide side but actually scared my father. To put it into perspective, other than snakes, nothing – and I mean nothing- scared my father.

It had started a normal day, cake for breakfast, no lunch and nothing but smiles. It was around the summer or spring time because I remember the windows being open and the smell of the fresh breeze always made me smile. I had one of those little red and white radio shack radios. You know, the ones with the little microphone.

This particular day, my little radio shack radio fell from the bookcase in my closet and stopped working. The day turned grisly once that happened. I attempted to fix the broken dream all on my own. I remember putting the little spring back on to close the cassette door and tightening the thin piece of metal that controlled the radio stations. However, no matter what I did- the antenna was still stuck inside and I hadn't the strength to pull it up.

I remember a panic and anger that just took me over. I started yelling until my father had called upstairs wondering what the matter was. I told him I was fine and it was nothing. He pressed on wonddering why I was yelling until finally I broke down and told him. More like screamed from the top of the stairs, little broken radio in hand, "MY RADIO IS BROKEN AND I CAN'T FIX IT. "

"Well give it to me and I'll fix it then", my father replied. Then suddenly, to make matters worse, I hurled the radio down the stairs at my father. I remember the look on his face, utter terror. He left me alone for the rest of the day but he was not mad at me, he simply didn't know how to respond. He didn't know how to help.

There were many more days like that as a child. There were many incidents where stuff got broken, people got hurt and words were said that could never be taken back. Now, mind you, I am a very sentimental person. Everything makes me cry or everything makes me say "aww". No joke. So you can understand why this next story still aches in my heart over thirty years later.

For my sixth birthday my sister picked out, all on her own, a Get-Along-Gang caboose to match the characters my mother had given me. She was so excited as I unwrapped the gift she just knew I would love. I noticed right away that the characters I had were not made for that patricular caboose but because she was so happy to give it to me I went along. I was just thrilled she took the effort. Imagine, my big sister was excited to give me a gift.

A few days later, sisters will be sisters and we were arguing over something so minute I cannot even remember. Needless to say, she had run down the stairs after attempting to get the last word. Immediately, without a single thought, I ran into my room, grabbed that little caboose and hurled it down the stairs (much like the little radio) and screamed, "I HATE THIS CABOOSE. IT'S NOT EVEN THE RIGHT ONE." And the little caboose shattered. Almost immediately I realized what I had done and ran down the stairs trying to put the pieces back together. All the while, crying hysterically because I broke something somebody got me. My sister got me. But as I learned through every heartache, the pieces don't always go back togther.

"I got the suitcase packed Penny"

As the years went by I perfected my competent appearance until everyone around me found me to be a highly energetic and happy individual without a care in the world. But still, the façade was exhausting to maintain and sometimes I just couldn't hide anymore and then people eventually left. All the while I put on my happy face and could coin the phrase, "I am fine".

"

I have given you reason to judge.

I have faltered a girl and conjured a burden

So avoid

"

Im Fine !!!.
Be Fine !!!.
Better be fine...
" Sumie whats wrong?"
" Nothing why

TRUST ME, I'M A LICENSED PSYCHIATRIST

As one would imagine, I've had a lot of doctors during my time on this Earth, and more of them shrinks than medical doctors. I never fully trusted any of them, minus a couple, and I especially liked to play with the awful ones. When I say 'play' I am referring to mind games on a shrink. You know what it's like to win a battle of wits against a shrink until she quite literally fires you. She stormed out of her office and the next thing I know my social worker was sitting beside me as the office looked to find me another one. The disappointment rang through the room, not only with the social worker and other doctors, but my parents that were sitting beside me in the waiting room. They were the most disappointed.

Anyhow, I never felt the need for a shrink because I could do it myself, take care of myself. The state, schools and parents felt otherwise. So, I would play with them, lie to them, make it a game.

The doctor that 'fired' me, well she started okay. Listening and "mmm hmmming" as shrinks often did but then she became quick to judge and instead of offering advise felt that given my age and issue that I should just listen to whatever she tells me to do. I don't think so. I lucked out in the end, and you're going to find me to be absolutely horrible for what I did next.

As luck would have it, she had a son who had killed himself a couple years prior. You want to get someone to passionately despise you rather quickly? Remind them of their dead son committing suicide because they were not a good enough shrink or parent to help them.

That's right, I did that, and felt horrible for doing so but I won my case and that woman would not be telling me what to do or feeding my parents advise anymore. After all, what is wrong with these people? I'm perfectly normal- just look at my smile.

Most of my shrinks were that way in one way or another. Although I did have a fiendishly sociopathic med prescriber who lost his license for borrowing money from patients and writing false prescriptions. He was a peach. He put me on such a heavy dose of Lithium I was almost toxic. It was not until momma- during one of her good weeks- walked into his office and demanded a script adjustment did he stop giving me the Lithium. Instead he gave me a sleeping pill, believing that all I needed was some sleep and I'd be normal. Well, a narcotic sleeping pill not intended for anyone with a certain illness like bi-polar puts that patient in an unconscious manic episode. I'm sure that did wonders for my overall mental health.

Then when I reached 18, I decided I did not need a doctor at all, or meds. That was the choice I was allowed to make. Looking back, I should have expected my parents to intervene, or at the very least say something. But momma was getting sicker at that time and felt that I was perfect the way I was, and dad would never intervene with such a thing. I still don't know if it was lack of caring or because he legitimately felt he had no right to say anything. Maybe a bit of both.

Don't get me wrong, a lot of the times I was great. A normal teenager. But other times, hospitalization and half-way houses for me. None of which my parents would visit. Although there was one time when I was about 19-20 that I had to move in with my father. When he was informed by the doctors and staff at the half-way house that it was recommended I have supervision for the next few days. he had other plans to go with his new girlfriend to our family in CT. He left me alone for the first day in a new apartment after spending weeks in the state hospital and then later half-way house. He just left me alone although he did leave me cash. Dad always proved his worth with cash. I guess it's a good thing I didn't need his help anyway.

If I was to count, I have probably gone through at least a dozen shrinks outside of the hospitals and only two of them- TWO- were worth a damn. Both well into my thirties and in the same office. After an incident (or episode as doctors sometimes refer to them as) I was informed by the hospital, of the regular medical kind, that they will have me committed next time they see me if I am not a patient of the local community mental health office. You see, as some of you with the same or similar diagnosis is aware, I am on the list as a "worst case scenarios". No standard, private shrink will take me with my diagnosis, so I'm left with one type of facility. This facility sees all kinds but all of which seem to be severe cases. Either way, they were willing and eager to help.

The first shrink they gave me was tough but effective. She played to my weaknesses like not being able to lose and wanting to appear normal. But she later went on to a different job and left me with one of the other facility doctors. This woman, what a nutjob. She was the flightiest, most unorganized individual I have ever seen in the health field of any kind. Fortunately for me she soon left the facility's employment and they paired me with my current shrink. For once in 36 years, I had someone on the other side of the desk who was passionate and understanding of my situation. As you have probably guessed, my diagnosis is grim meaning I am stuck with it for the rest of my life, and no amount of medication or treatment will take that away. But my current doctor takes the time to individualize my treatment and even though I may never be healed, I can cope better with the situation and move on.

She convinced me to finally partake in DBT or Dialectical Behavior Therapy. For almost 20 years I was hesitant on DBT because I feared it a waste of time and ineffective. In my early, early, twenties I refused to partake merely because the way it was sold to me was a means of making myself more tolerable to normies (normies is the coined phrase for those individuals not mentally ill in a couple of the institutions that fluffed my pillow). But that isn't it at all. DBT is a way to control your emotions and make some things in life, and those stressful situations more tolerable. I'm quite pleased to have finally decided to join a DBT group and it was a decision well-worth it.

For once, there's a group of 'like minded' individuals who can teach me tricks of the trade and who have similar situations and fears. Each week I get to sit around a table (always in my same spot of course) and be honest and open without the fear of persecution or ridicule. We can learn from each other and we can be comfortable in our own skin. For those individuals questioning if DBT is right for you, I would highly recommend it.

If there is anything to be taken from this small bit on the endless world of shrinks it is this. There are good ones out there that will take the time to not blindly earn your trust but willingly accept that your trust must be rightfully earned. Myself and others in similar situations don't need someone to feel what we feel or live how we live, because it won't happen. We need doctors that will tell us, "this fucking sucks for you. I can't take away what happened to you. I can't take away your illness, but I can hopefully make it more bearable". I urge every one of you to tell your doctors that, especially the new ones. Tell them that's what you want to hear and once they acknowledge you can't be cured but you CAN be helped then you can sit your ass down in the chair and start talking.

Now that brings us to another uncomfortable but messy topic, institutions. Large, small, windowed, or manicured lawns, they are all the same building at the end of the day. They are the walls keeping the crazies from the normies.

Side note: I urge you to read through my short story at the end of this book called "They Call Me Tiff".

THE UGLY TRUTH ABOUT MENTAL HOSPITALS

Mental institutions started popping up in the early 19th century when counties or families were no longer able to care for their loved ones (or the local crack-pot). We have all heard of facilities like Athens Lunatic Asylum and Danvers State hospital where diagnosis and treatment were not only outrageous but barbaric. The science available to doctors at the time warranted such treatment but the fact of the matter is, the idea of the mental institution is forever tainted with these archaic pasts

Much has changed since then. Certain archaic treatments are obviously no longer utilized, and a husband cannot just ship his wife away to an asylum because divorce is against his religious beliefs.

To be honest, there probably isn't much ugly- actual-truth to the rumors behind present day institutions. Typically, the privately funded ones are very clean, and the staff is very nice, and the state hospitals are a 180-degree turnaround from the private ones but that seems to be caused by being understaffed and underfunded.

Don't get me wrong, every time I have been in one, I wanted nothing more than to escape its evil grasp but that's because the nature of the visit and the fact that it was always against my will.

Brookside in NH was my first and third stint at a mental institution. That one was worse than most but still not all that bad. I'm sure you have staff somewhere abusing patients and hospitals somewhere that are dirty and unkept but don't judge them all this way. They aren't all what you see based in horror movies and crime shows. Should you ever find yourself in one, the chances of getting killed are slim to none.

So, on one side, you have the privately funded hospitals like Brookside. When I first went to Brookside, I was very little and when my parents told me I was going to a hospital I figured I was getting tests done or seeing a surgeon about my feet. Not a chance. I remember pulling up the long drive in the back of momma's caravan and seeing this beautiful building that looked like a storybook mansion.

I remember going through the big doors and momma was crying. After that, the only thing I remembered was watching cartoons on the television when they handed out meds. I don't recall what I was on then, but it couldn't have been too bad because I was so young. Although it did mellow me out so I would assume something comparable to a Valium.

The second stint, when I was a bit older, fourth or fifth grade, was at another privately funded hospital in Hampstead. That stay I remember a bit better given my age but still nothing severe. I was only there for a couple of weeks until I was able to work the doctor into letting me return home. I wouldn't see the state hospital for a few years, well into my late teens, but I did get to stay at Brookside again a few years later when I was a freshman in high school.

My boyfriend at the time convinced my dad to have me meet with the school counselor and later an outside doctor once he found out I stopped taking my medication. My parents tricked me saying that I was getting an 'outpatient evaluation' only to have me committed again.

This time I was old enough to be so angry. Angry at my parents and angry at my boyfriend. This stay I remember quite well. I remember my parents walking with the doctor to drop me at Ward B. I remember not saying a word to anyone. I had never been so angry. I also remember the double doors to the ward shutting and my parents discussing where to go have lunch- never looking back.

That stint at Brookside was also short lived before I convinced my dad I was normal and to take me home. I played with his weakness of wanting a 'normal' daughter. But in the short time there I was able to meet my very first Sociopath, not one to mess with and to this day the most feared person (or group of people) I know. She tried to kill her parents by setting the house on fire because they would not let her go to a party. We were informed by the doctors that we were to talk with her as little as possible and most certainly avoid telling her what's 'wrong' with us. A more appropriate coin for the same meaning, 'our diagnosis'.

At this time, I also had my first crush on a doctor, unfortunately he wasn't my doctor, but I did get the opportunity to stare often without him noticing. I also broke my first nose although did not intend to and later felt terrible. I could not look the orderly in the eye until he had approached me first. This orderly with the once perfect nose lost a grip on my legs after they gave me a tranquilizer shot. What happens when someone is given a tranquilizer is not what you'd assume. For the first few seconds the tranquilized individual has the strength of a house and when he lost his grip, I managed to kick him clear in the nose, although there was no intended target in mind. Lucky shot!

Years later, I found myself at the state hospital and that stay was much different but still most the same. They didn't give me a roommate because of something regarding my sleep, I don't remember although I was grateful for not having to deal with just one more person. The stay was mild except they kept me more medicated than I was used to. Probably due to staffing issues. Medicated folks have a tendency not to fight.

The one thing I hated most about the hospital, ECT. For those of you who don't know, ECT is Electroconvulsive Therapy. Think shock treatment as you've seen on TV but a lot cleaner and you're anesthetized. They believe by giving the patient a seizure the brain is reset and the psychotic symptoms are cured. It works for a little while but those of us with bipolar are STILL bipolar. You lose your short-term memory for a few days and then the problem just comes right back.

As an adult, upon leaving the hospitals they often put you in a half-way or rehabilitation/ transition home. Typically, these weren't too bad, mostly like living back with your parents as kids when you had specific dinner time and rules- like don't kill the other patients. And typically, they weren't co-ed. In fact, I don't think I stayed in any of the co-ed ones. That would've just ended in sex. That's what I do.

There was one home that I really liked. Well "liked" is relative in comparison to the other places I had been. The doctors and staff were few and they didn't treat you as a mental patient. They didn't scoff every time I needed a cigarette because they had to escort me outside. In fact, one of the orderlies smoked. A lot. He would come get me from my room or the common area every time he went outside to smoke. He bought me a pack when I was out and would even pick me up cottage cheese at the gas station down the street when I wouldn't eat because I didn't like the food the hospital sent over. I believe I already told you that I'm stubborn.

"

The broken tiles look down on me

I crawl from the depths just so I can see

The broken walls looking up at me

Now that I am untamed and free

Both down and up, up and down

Scenes keep changing

But always run down.

Looking out, through crooked bars

From a crooked floor

Looking out at crooked stars

"

EVERY PAIR OF NEW SHOES MEANT A NEW MAN

I went through relationships like I did jobs up until I found the right one in both. My relationships never ended well and as you can imagine they weren't the standard teen angst devastation. My devastation meant scars, teeth and lots of alcohol. Only to realize three days later that such commotion was not necessary when you're young and cute and you had already found a replacement.

Don't get me wrong, every relationship EVERY ONE. I noticed somethings about myself during the horrific break-up stage that I would vouge to later fix with the next one so this whole ordeal could never happen again. It always did happen again, and again, and again. It did not matter how many times I tell myself "don't do it, they'll get fed up and leave you". You'll see from my current relationship (after the few older ones listed below) I am meant to push them out the door and they are meant to leave me.

Another thing you should be made aware of as I drag you through bits of the longest of those relations is that I started very young. Sometimes I wish that my relationships didn't start SO young but let's face it I could've made that decision back then.

Let's start off with Joe. Joe was my biggest crush since I was a girl much younger than eleven (when he first found me attractive), but he was over eight years my senior. When I was eleven, Joe was nineteen… and he was perfect. Well, to me anyhow but perfect all the same. Long flowing hair, green on the sides and blonde in the middle. When he wore it in a mohawk it even looked more dashing- as momma would say. He had tattoos and was the ultimate bad-boy. But Joe had issues if you didn't already determine by the whole eleven- nineteen thing.

Let me draw you more of a backstory here. Every Summer I would spend at least a few weeks to a month in Syracuse with momma's family. Joe and his sister Cheria were my aunt's neighbors for years, and each year as I grew older, I found myself more infatuated with Joe. He was a gorgeous specimen if I had known what that truly was so young. As luck would have it, I was good friends with his little sister who was close to my age. I would always tag along when he took Cheria to the mall or the movies. Once I was able to even sit next to him and hold his arm at the scary movie. Well, shortly after that blessed move union, tragedy struck. Joe's dad had stormed off one evening drunker than one who could barely walk let alone drive and he had taken Cheria with him. He did not die, but the same could not be said for her. She was thrown from the car and died almost instantly, the one saving grace for such a horrific event.

Joe's mother couldn't take the loss of her beloved youngest and the beast she called lover sitting in jail – which was the least he deserved. One Christmas Eve about a year and half later she drank herself into such a raging depression that she felt it best to shoot herself and leave her thirteen-year-old son alone with no parents, no sister, no prospects. I guess something flipped in Joe that day and he was never the same person again. The smile you could count on and the silly laugh all but disappeared. He was broken.

But from that point on Joe took care of me. I must have filled the missing piece in his heart after Cheria passed because he would keep tabs on me all year until I would visit again and then he would teach me things like how to jump a train and skip stones across the reservoir. Then one night when I was 11, I struck a more curious note within him. He suddenly looked at me differently. He would suddenly watch the other boys around me as if to pounce should they make a move. In his own disturbed way, he loved me.

The night I lost my virginity wasn't something out of a fairytale like all girls suspect. All of us, my cousins, a couple of friends and myself had been planning to sleep on the bank between the train tracks and the reservoir. This was a common occurrence at least a few nights out of my time in Syracuse so I didn't suspect that night would have been any different. I was pleasantly mistaken and that night became the night I would remember for the rest of my life.

At the last-minute Joe decided to come and join us. I thought It surprising given that he never had in the past and that he was older than all of us. Nevertheless, part of me was thrilled to be sleeping near him as he always made me feel safe.

For the most part, the night had pretty much gone as planned. There was lots of drinking, smoking and hooking up. I was the youngest of us all so while my cousin and my friend Lori were tag teaming what they considered to be the "hottest guy in their high school", I sat by the fire burning leaves and watching the sparks fly into the air and dissipate before reaching ground again as ash. It always amazed me how the most beautiful spark jut fizzled out into nothingness. Depressing ash. That's how I was beginning to feel that night watching everyone around me, depressing ash. Was there ever that fizzling spark in me?

Joe was deep in video game conversation with the second oldest of us, my friend Casey. I kept peeking over his way in between fizzles and quite a few times caught him peering back. I finally got up the nerve to go swimming in the dark by myself to try and liven up my mood. Swimming always managed to do that for me. I decided to tell Joe just in case anyone was looking for me and not surprising his response, "not by yourself you don't" and he bid adieu to his conversation with Casey and followed me over to the boat launch which was the easiest way to avoid the rocks that lined the lake.

I playfully argued with him about coming with me before flirtingly telling him he was allowed to join me as long as his clothes stayed at the launch. To my surprise there was no hesitation. I remember, clear as day, watching him take down his shorts and just stand there in front of me. I must have looked a fool but that's when I realized that I was now someone that was more to him than just his lost sister's friend.

I was too embarrassed to take off my own clothes so before he could argue I ran past him straight into the water and started to swim away. I didn't know what any of this actually meant. I didn't know what I was supposed to do next. Joe was generally very well liked and very calm headed and now here he was, naked in the water with someone eight years his junior. What was I supposed to do next?

Before I could even gather my bearings, he caught up to me in the water and wrapped his legs around my waist so I couldn't swim away. And then he kissed me. He grabbed my chin to pull me forward and just kissed me. I had been kissed before, but never like this. Never the more experienced,

46

gentle kiss. And that's when he said it. "I love you dragonfly."

Dragonfly was his nickname for me for as long as I can remember. In many cultures, dragonflies symbolized lightness and the ability to adapt. He agreed with momma that there was a light inside of me that could brighten up even the darkest of spaces and when that light grew dim the darkness around me would grow at an alarming rate. When Joe kissed me and said the magical words that little girls love to hear I imagine that light grew ten times brighter. To this day I believe Joe had love for me in his own way, but not how it played out that night.

Still unaware of what to do next, I decided to go on instinct. I started to swim ashore in hopes that he would follow. Which of course he did. Before I could grab my towel, he wrapped his arms around my waist and kissed me yet again. This time longer and more fervent. He started to pull down my wet clothes and kiss up and down, my shoulders and neck and then moved his way down to the other, more private areas. Before he landed on the sand, naked and wet.

I was becoming more aware of what was expected of me and I followed suit arriving next to him, on the sand and now naked as well. Before I could politely reject or let alone react in any ladylike manner, he was leaning over me. I won't go much further into any detail but I'm sure you can determine the next steps that were taken. Before I knew it, my virginity was gone. Naked and wet on the sand. On the reservoir bank. In Syracuse. Hundreds of miles from home.

So, when people tell me that Joe was a creep and a pedophile, I can't believe it. He didn't go after me until many

47

years later. He went after me because I was the closest thing to his sister, and I looked like an eighteen-year-old myself. What we shared that drunken night on the reservoir bank certainly didn't mean a whole lot, but it meant something because of who he was. So, I urge you to look at that relationship for what it was and not the age difference- and what that means. Joe was kind to me, and I looked up to him for his ability to move on. He was troubled, yes. I don't deny that. But if I had to lose my virginity at that young an age, I wouldn't have chosen anyone else, my age or not.

For years after that I had the itty-bitty little middle school relationships and it was very hard to convince boys to have sex. I was cute but we were all so young so they'd be interested but scared shitless. Imagine being a woman nowadays and having to seek sex out. It doesn't happen, after a certain age sex will always find you.

Then cut to eighth grade. My eighth-grade beau was a tall Italian with piercing blue eyes. Another bad boy if you could imagine. John was all the 'good girl's' dream. He was as charming as you could be at that age always riding around on his bike and whatnot. He was their bad boy dream, but I got him. Originally, I never planned on going out with John even though he'd been trying. I wanted to keep him as a friend- and a backup- from my boyfriend Mike. Always remember to have a backup, and for good reason. Mike broke up with me out of nowhere one day because I quote "you are a crazy bitch". Oh, if only he truly knew. But John knew. We had that friendship where we knew everything about each other- and he wanted me anyway. So, the same day I broke up with Mike I started going out with John.

But that relationship ended up not being everything I had imagined, and we broke up after about a year. Now cue the remainder of high school. About two weeks after breaking up with John I met Chris.

Chris was something to behold. Some girls were after him because he was a bad boy (but not like John) but he was sweeter than you could imagine and no matter how bad I treated him- he loved me. Throughout our relationship he saw me in and out of hospitals, changing meds, changing doctors and sleeping with everyone anytime he went on vacation with his family. Against the better wishes of his family we stayed together for almost four years until I finally got sick of cheating and just found someone to replace him with.

But I didn't just "pull off the band aid" and break up with him. I was afraid that his replacement wouldn't amount to anything so I asked him if we could take a two-week break. He waited almost two months before I told him, "no, this isn't going to work out." He waited, without finding a replacement himself, for me to screw around and then leave him out of nowhere.

But the almost four years we were together were amazing (well, as amazing as a highschool relationship could be). He ended up being my best friend for a while and I relied on him for everything. Companionship, secret keeping, sexy male nurse- all of it. What I did to him was unforgiveable. He knew me and he loved me anyway. He hated my meds but loved how they kept me safe. I had done nothing to deserve him sticking around, but he did. If I was to tell him anything, I'd say "I'm sorry for all of it- every bit- and if it's any comfort, you dodged a bullet when I left you for Jay- I'm still a crazy bitch."

Then cue Jay, another bad boy. Are you catching the theme yet? Jay was definitely not Chris, but I thought he was hot, and I was apparently sick of Chris for some reason. Jay couldn't handle me. The day I had my first complete mental breakdown was with Jay. I had picked him up from work at the mall and got into it with him about my thoughts of him cheating. One thing led to another and I ended up slitting my wrist during an episode. He just punched me in the side of the face and stepped out of the car. At that point, I was having a full-blown mental breakdown. He didn't respond the way I wanted him to, and he wouldn't get back in the car. He didn't go for help. In fact, he never talked to me again. This monstrous relationship went on for about two years and then wouldn't you know who came to my rescue when I got shipped away to a halfway house but Chris. Yes, that Chris, He was in a new relationship, but I needed him, so he came.

After I got out of the Mill House, I went to live with my father in his two-bedroom apartment in Derry. No boyfriend, hardly any friends and stitches on my arms and wrist. I was quite the catch but just a few days after moving in with dad I met Jeff.

Jeff was not a bad boy by any means, but he was a death metalist with an amazing guitar skill and long curly hair. I was ready for the new and nice or so I thought. He was so kind to me and I chewed him alive! Although some of the issues did revolve around his mother who I think had a very unnatural obsession with her son.

One time when we were having sex in his bedroom, he got a call on the house phone. Well, his mother, knowing

50

what we were doing, walks in the room to hand him the phone and then when he told her to take a message because he was naked, she insisted he get up and grab the phone. That was just one of many creepy, obsessive, overall disturbing occurrences.

About two and a half years later, she won. I hadn't seen him in about four days, and he was supposed to be taking me back to my dorm room when out of nowhere she tells him he needs to drive her home. Well, I lost it. I had just had it with that woman. He left me! And then wouldn't even come outside to talk to me. He knew I was sick, and I didn't handle that kind of rejection well. He left me for his mother and then had the audacity to not even come outside and talk to me as his mother sat inside gloating, waiting for her ride.

After Jeff there were several more rather short relationships ranging from one to about eight or nine months and then I hooked up with shithead, oh I'm sorry. Let's call him Wayne. I'd say that Wayne was my punishment for all the terrible misgivings of previous relationships, but I don't even know that fate would deem it even. Wayne was dreadful, he was a beating, lazy, money stealing loser. I used to have to rent him video games in the morning if I wanted to hang out with any girlfriends because it was my duty to entertain him. He gave Tennessee citizens a bad name and to this day I will never date a guy from Tennessee. He used my illnesses to his advantage. He would steal something from me and tell me that I gave it away or he would beat me and tell me that I hit first, or it was all in my mind.

There was one particular incident when he nearly killed me. It wasn't until he hurt my cat Zachary that I fought back. When the police asked me, "Do you want to press charges?" I said "no". Why would I say no? A sane person, a normie, would most likely scream "Yes" for the world to hear that you were putting that psycho where he belongs. That's what I should have said, instead of "no".

I always told myself I would never stay with someone abusive and could never fathom how some of these women I heard about did. It's easy, I used to think. Just leave! Not so easy. I tried to leave him once and he reminded me that he knew where my young niece and nephew lived and they trusted him to open the door. Finally, I had the opportunity to get rid of him, in fact I did. He got shipped back to Tennessee and well, because I can't be alone. I deemed it worth dealing with him until I found something better. A replacement. So, I had him move back. Fortunately, after a little over three years with him, I met my ex-husband. His replacement.

In fact, I had my first double date scheduled with my ex-husband the day shithead was back to Tennessee for the last time.

My ex- Kevin is another means of me needing karma to bite me in the ass. The man worshiped me. Sick me, fat me, ugly me, me with the flu. There was nothing I could do that would make that man think that I wasn't amazing. And even though he wasn't my type, more of a homebody, he was an amazing man. To this day, I'm engaged to another and I will always say he was nothing short of amazing. And, to this day I will tell you that I wish I could say he was an asshole because then I wouldn't come across as being such a bitch.

Kevin and I dated for about two years and were married for almost seven. I actually did pretty well being married to Kevin even though according to my therapist I hit a 'depressive state' for about six of the seven years I was married. I'd have to say for the most part though I maybe had an episode every couple of months instead of ferocious episodes about every other day. I'm not sure if it was the depressive episode or simply Kevin's reaction to me, or maybe the fact that I whole heartedly trusted him not to cheat. The man made it very clear that he adored me so why would he cheat. If I look back on all my relationships him and Chris were the only ones to look at me a certain way, react to my episodes a certain way, even something as simple as talk to me a certain way.

Well, like every relationship, all things were naturally going to come to an end. I decided about six years into our marriage that I wanted something different- like I had so many times before. I ended up having an affair right under his nose with a good friend of mine. Not just cheating this time, a full-blown falling in love affair. Even when I admitted to the affair he still stayed. I had the affair for two reasons. The first being the obvious, I was bored and the second as an 'out' in my marriage. Kevin insisted I could do anything, and he would forgive me or forget it, except cheat. I not only cheated but had an affair and expected him to call it quits. I never can- it always needs to be them.

But he didn't call it quits. Instead he told me that he couldn't give me up. I was just too amazing. Amazing? Seriously?? I am anything but. I'm a psychotic bitchy mess who cheats on quite literally everybody. That is not the picture of amazing. That's the picture of crazy. So, then it was up to me to call it quits. To give up. Something I've only done once before. Even when they beat me. The only reason that ended was because my parents took care of it. Imagine being twenty-four and your parents move you into their

53

house and tell shithead- I mean Wayne- that he needs to go back to Tennessee.

After separating from Kevin, I hooked up with a long-time friend who I'm still with today. Almost three years and I've only cheated on him three times and accuse him of cheating every day. Seth and I met back in 2001 and had sex for a good solid year and a half after that. When I questioned him about us being together, he told me he could not handle me. Apparently now he thinks he can. I don't believe it. He doesn't react to me how I would like and there is obviously a reason I accuse him of cheating even though he insists that the only one unfaithful is me. But, since 2001 he is quite literally the only man I want affection from or can cuddle with.

All the relationships and all the men, I would be damned if they tried to curl up next to me in bed. As it is the only other man, I could even sleep next to was my ex-husband but even he wasn't allowed to touch me in my sleep. But Seth, him I want nothing more than to lay on his chest in the middle of the night or have him lay behind me and hold me tight.

But like I said, he doesn't react like Kevin or Chris. He seems to have grown almost fed up with the episodes and when I need a fight- and he knows it- he refuses to. Is this the way it's supposed to be? Are people not supposed to react but instead just listen to me scream and throw stuff. Even when I scream in his face or push him, he just walks away and makes me chase after him.

My doctors tell me that is an acceptable response, but I can't believe it. He's almost had me hospitalized ten times by now and again my doctors tell me that he can provide necessary evidence and quite frankly, hospitalization would be the desirable outcome. How can I love- and need- a man so much that it feels my life would crumble without him when he doesn't give me what I need? What most of them have always given me. Instead, nothing.

Why is it that I blame – and have terrible thoughts about- him cheating with no discernible evidence when I am the one with undeniable evidence of cheating against me? Is that the reason? Is it because I've cheated with precisely every relationship? Or is it that I'm so afraid to lose him?

We may never know. Until then we are engaged to be married, I still blame him for cheating with no grounds, and until recently was providing episodic cinema almost every night. Oh, the episodes... the dreaded and shameful episodes.

ONE EPISODE, TWO EPISODES, THREE EPISODES, FOUR

For those of you that suffer with what therapists either call 'episodic behavior' or 'symptomatic behavior' you are not alone. I would have to guess that millions of us out there quite frankly lose their minds ever so often when the meds fail at their jobs. And fail miserably at that.

"You had one job"

My symptoms came early, and like a hailstorm. Little five-year-old me was not educated or wise enough to understand what was happening. What it meant when the mind completely broke- busted off its hinges.

I don't remember much of my first episode, but I know it came quick, worked it's magic quick and swiftly went away leaving a series of broken toys and burned hands in its path. I remember the feeling after it all happened, not right before, but after. You have this overwhelming feeling of shame without recollection as to why. You knew something happened. You knew you got mad. Yet, you didn't feel yourself amp up out of control for little to no reason. My reaction was not warranted by the small amount of trouble that was caused for me.

I take you now to my teens. Full of teen angst and morose hormones as it was- bring in Borderline and Bipolar symptoms. Bring in the inability to recognize emotions let alone control them. Some of what I would consider episodes I imagine were not simply because I still knew what I was doing. I still had control. But because I didn't fully understand the diseases yet I would blame 'episodic behavior' on many of my 'plain bitch' moments. I imagine It was so I could feel less shameful of anything I may have done to hurt people. After all, it's easier to excuse sick than mean. And I got mean!

Nevertheless, episodes did exist and got me hospitalized, or lost my friends, made my parents cry. The worst. The feelings of the episodes were much more intense as I got older. Unfortunately, I'm able to remember most of the them. Except of course for the midst of the episode when I don't remember much. Imagine your body being taken over and spouting every possible mean thing you could think of to your closest friends and family. Imagine the body snatcher hitting, scratching and biting those around you. Also, imagine if you will taking razors or cigarettes and marking your body beyond repair. These parts I truly don't remember or have much control of.

However, as the episode starts to wind down, you do feel, you do know. But you can't quite stop yet. That's when the pain from the cuts or burns, any of the new scars, starts to surface. When you grab your hair and just want to rip it out because your mind just won't stop. Imagine again the hailstorm but this time you're stuck in the middle and your body is covered in burns and cuts. Every bit of hale just blasts through you, opening any dormant pain receptacle.

The worse part of it all- the whole wind down- is the look on other people's faces. The body snatcher rode through like a hurricane and the loved ones around you were right in its path. Each of them would adorn looks that screamed, "we want to forgive you but what you did. What you said, is completely unforgiveable". Immediately you fill with shame.

57

On top of the mistaken mind and racing thoughts- you now have shame. Absolute. And you must live with that forever.

Now let me bring you to present day. I'm currently in my late thirties and have become aware of what my diseases mean and so familiar with the episodes that I can feel them coming. I can't quite stop them all the time, but know they are here. No matter how much I learn about the diseases and about this episodic behavior it doesn't make it any easier.

Episodes come as harsh and fast as a tidal wave, and they fizzle out just the same. I have dread before they've even come and gone because I know what I'm about to do. For those of you symptomatic that can relate- for the dread you feel, I am truly sorry and for those of you who can't relate and are merely reading these accounts to get a base of reference or to try and understand- you never will. Words cannot describe the agony. As years went by the episodes got stronger and the anguish in the beginning and end worsened each time.

I'm not sure that I portrayed properly what it feels like to have an episode so here's another stab at it. Hopefully this will help you understand a little but more at what we go through.

"Way to go Sue"

Imagine if you will my fiancé and I are having a tiff over his cheating, or lack of proof for, and I can feel myself start to shake and warm up. Next thing I know, he walks away from me because I've started to yell, and I storm after him. I'm screaming and crying so loud that my voice is breaking, and the shaking worsens. I start to pick up anything of his that I can reach and throw it around. Now cue my voice, louder and even more shaky. My entire body trembles and tightens as if a negative 30 wind has just burst freezing air right through me.

I put my hands to my knees and bend over, half to limit the pain on my joints, half to keep myself from falling over. I start to scream something like "I HATE YOU. I HATE YOU. GONE.YOU GOT TO GO. TAKE YOUR SKANK WITH YOU- SHE'S WAITING." My voice is almost maniacal as I start to laugh and cry and laugh some more.

I can feel my nose dripping down my chin (which sticks out a little so it makes a nice boarding zone) and I start to rake my fingernails across my cheeks mumbling nonsense to myself. I run from room to room finding more stuff to throw mumbling hysterically. Things like "you'll get yours. Karma will get you. Go fuck your skank. Karma will get you."

My head will start to hurt, and my skin starts to crawl with an uneasy chill. I pull at my hair as I wander the apartment now looking for something to cut myself with. Something to make it stop. There's no reason, there's no power. The voice that tells you eventually that you need to stop is still muffled by the blood rushing to your brain. You are in physical pain and mental anguish and you quite literally have no control.

Other times I have had episodes against either strangers or mere acquaintances- which offers even less satisfaction when you are amped up. There was one time I was so sick of my nasty downstairs neighbors parking in my second parking spot that I immediately amped up. And the non-confrontational side makes the simple passive aggressive look like a bull in a china shop.

I could immediately feel myself warming up. Like a burning sensation that starts at the feet and works its way to your ears. Running through the apartment I grabbed the loudest most thumping speaker I could find and placed it right over their living room. I blared death metal so loud that the people down the street probably heard. As if that wasn't enough, I started jumping up and down right over where their kitchen and dining room were. I got my point across but nearly had a stroke doing it. They moved that car and moved it quick, but left me with no satisfaction because now these people probably thought I was crazy

When I was little, I would beg the gods or other powers that be to warn me when the episodes were coming. Now I beg the same powers to take that foresight from me. Let me just run my path, do my harm and move on. Only allow me such dread one time- at the end. At the face in the crowd, at the smashed belongings, at all the blood that escaped my body when it was not my own.

The more episodes I had the more scars formed and the more a piece of me was ripped apart by the shame and guilt of what I became. What I am.

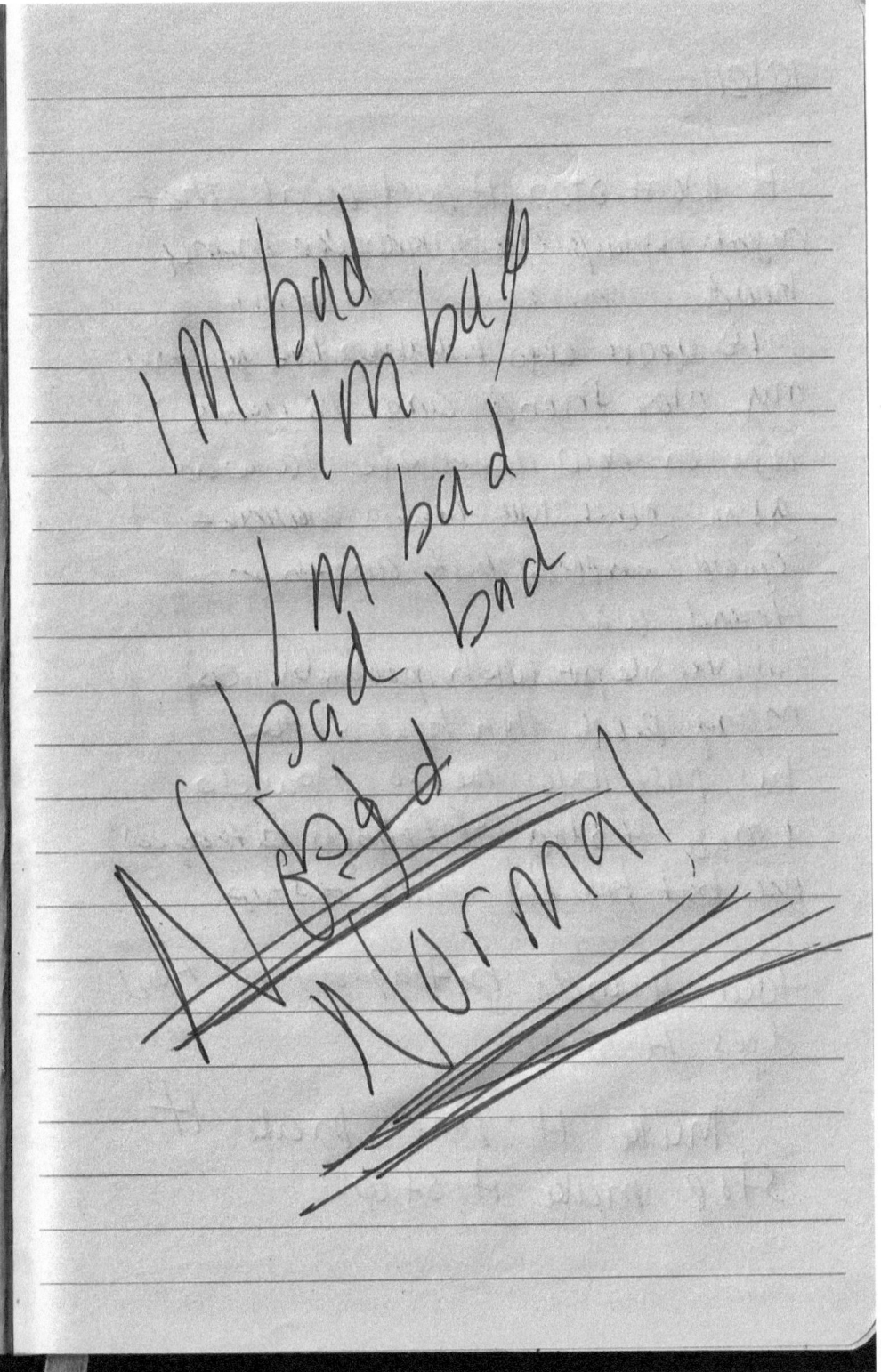

AND WHEN I'M NOT IN AN EPISODE

Cognitive distortions are described as "an exaggerated or irrational thought pattern." Exaggerated or irrational. Let's break this down a bit more shall we.

Exaggerated is described as "represented as larger, better or worse than in reality". "Worse than in reality" is the epitome of what makes borderlines- borderlines, at least in my opinion. If something is there one day, you have it. If that same thing is moved from one place to another the next day- then you don't have it.

In my case, and current relationship with Seth as best an example. Worse is life. It's the bread and butter of my day. Please don't think I am a person full of hatred and dread- I am quite the opposite. But I am doom and gloom with a smile on my face. When I pass someone in the hallway and offer them a big and bright "how are you?" and they greet me back in exchange with a grunted "hello" stands to reason that person obviously hates me. Turns out those people are rarely greeting me that way out of scorn but simply because they are having a bad day.

When Seth calls me two minutes late or sounds like he's rushing to get me off the phone- the reason could very well be harmless. But what I think, cue the hailstorm, is that he's getting me off the phone to have a conversation with another woman whom he plans on bringing home. Two minutes! Two minutes turns to cheating. Now I know how silly that sounds or outrageous that makes me but it's what it seems to be. It seems to be the truth in my head so it must be. Even though now I'm sitting here, typing to you, telling you that I recognize it's outrageous, I still think it. I still think, outrageously, that two minutes late calling me couldn't possibly mean he was getting his coat on or caught in the hallways for a joke. He was two minutes late because he's cheating. Worse than reality!

Cognitive distortions are a matter of an irrational thought pattern. We've covered the exaggerated. Now this one's challenging because no matter how much I can recognize exaggerated; I can't recognize the irrational side. At least not enough to curb the thought and move on. And quite honestly, I'm far too stubborn to admit my thoughts were irrational when I'm in a rational mind. That would admit being wrong. I don't like being wrong- it makes me feel incompetent and less than. So, I will always drill the irrational thoughts into the subject matter. Typically, in my case that's Seth- who has stuck around from kids to engagement.

I will scream at him and hit him to make him recognize that what I'm saying must be truth. I've already 'exaggerated' the subject matter so let's bring It home. You are cheating! You are making a fool out of me! You are…. You are…. You are!

Types of cognitive distortions range from catastrophizing to the black and white thinking previously mentioned where there are no grays, no in between. Everything is to the extreme. For instance, Seth and I have a very above-average sex life but if there's ever a day he's not in the mood- then he's never in the mood and we never have sex.

Another type of cognitive distortion is a mental filter which disqualifies all good reactions, words, etcetera in a

63

situation and focusses on something less positive or hurtful. A good example of this is one day, while at the office, my boss had said he wishes I had handled a situation a certain way. Well now, even though in my rational mind I know I am very good at my job- everything I do has the potential to disappoint. More than a potential I'd say but an assumption that I will handle things incorrectly and disappoint my bosses.

Similarly, from my work life cue an "always being right" distortion. This is one of the issues I have in most every part of my life as well. Imagine if you will two bits of an argument. The correct one which is mine and the other loser faction. As much as it pains me to say, I am not always right, but I cannot stop. I would argue that the sky is pink until one of us strokes out or they just admit the sky is pink and go about their day. This is one of the cognitive distortions I found which is most often made readily available to those around me and in fact, giving them reason to judge. It's simple really. I cannot physically and mentally be wrong!

This brings us to one of my least favorite cognitive distortions, emotional reasoning. Emotional reasoning is the acceptance as one's emotions as fact. I take you back to the aforementioned 'bad thoughts'. I feel that Seth might be cheating so he obviously is. I also feel that he's mean when he fights with me during an episode, so it must be true. Of all the cognitive distortions, and there are many, this one tends to hurt me the most.

In the heat of the moment, I've heard some nasty things come from the mouths of my boyfriends, fiancés, etcetera. Some of these things include, bitch, crazy, psycho and my favorite, "you need to be in the hospital." Now we all say things in that heat of the moment we don't mean and they typically hurt. For me the crazy and the hospital are the worst things one can say and probably the only things you can't take back. Those things stick with me, and they haunt me.

So cognitive distortions are basically the equivalent of an episode while not experiencing complete episodic behavior. And often they stay with you, and they hurt. Sometimes, it seems to me, that the underlying difference between cognitive distortions and full-blown episodes is the amount of hair you pull out. My therapist once told me something brilliant when we were discussing my fiancés cheating without any proof. I told Seth that I wanted him to prove he WASN'T cheating and her response to that was simple. And rational. And logical. She said, "you can't disprove a negative".

"

These lies I've learned are my own.

Fantasies you can't break

Mine- own eyes have cracked

Revealing beneath

This dream to escape

When I'm awake

Tight- forever tight I'll hold on

Without proof or fact

These lies I've learned are my own

You cannot take them

Stop with your reasons

Let Judgement carry

You cannot take them

They're mine

"

THE LITTLE GIRL IN THE MIRROR AND OTHER FANCY SYMPTOMS

Another fun issue to overcome for many of us, psychotic symptoms. I am told that my psychotic symptoms come mainly from the bipolar side of things, which makes them more prevalent but borderlines experience symptoms as well when things have gone too far. The symptoms suffered differ from person to person and originally, I thought mine would be lumped up there with hallucinations. Turns out they are not; most of my issues are illusions.

One particular illusion is a little girl screaming at me. Imagine if you will, looking through a rear-view mirror and seeing people or things looking back at you. That's my illusion. And she has not one nice thing to say. This has been ongoing during some of the more intense episodes for as long as I can remember. Fortunately, I know she's not real and she's not actually there- just a sticker on my rearview- but a psychotic symptom, nonetheless. So, I know when she's showing her ugly head, I am either having a 'break' or about to.

Other illusions I have faced prior to a break are an old man, cartoon-like, with a big head telling me that I could be his daughter if I wanted to. Also, another little girl, a bit older than the more prevalent rude one but she doesn't do anything but cry. I focus on her and it looks as though she's about to give me a half-smile but then she just places her head in her hands and starts crying uncontrollably. I would've loved to have her smile back at me, that would have been a welcome illusion to see.

These illusions I face are unquestionably chilling. Not because they themselves are frightening sights or threatening really in any way but because I know what they stand for. When they show themselves it does not mean that I am frightened, it means I'm broken. It means my brain has got up and moved on without reality. They show up and Susie is broken, again.

The buzzing on the other hand, normal everyday life. Nobody ever thinks of hearing sounds as a hallucination but auditory hallucinations I would imagine are as prevalent as any other. Anyway, I digress, the buzzing is a daily occurrence also for as long as I can remember. I can hear other noises around me perfectly fine, but it seems as though the buzzing is the only thing allowing me to focus. It quite literally sounds like the buzz of a generator, faint but rhythmic, and in my head.

There was a time in high school when the doctor (the one that lost his license for borrowing money) medicated me with a drug, and I can't remember what the name was, that turned off the buzzing. My life was in ruin. I realized that I required that buzzing to focus, to concentrate, to even walk straight it would seem. I immediately stopped taking the medicine against my doctor's better wishes.

All-in-all I am quite lucky that my psychotic episodes aren't worse than they are. There are those of us out there that live every day wondering if something exists, or thinking they smell fire everywhere they go, and they are panic-stricken each day for their entirety. And although these episodic illusions are easily dealt with there are many other episodic behaviors that aren't so calm. For me, it's the maladaptive behavior. To put it bluntly, the cutting and burning my damn self.

I had started hurting myself as early as five and at that time it was mainly burning myself with momma's lighter or using the door frame in my bedroom to scratch myself until I bled. I didn't quite understand it at that young an age and not sure I fully understand It now.

The interpretations of why I hurt myself were always given TO me so I assumed throughout the years that they all understood more than me and what they believed must have been truth. They came up with all kinds of interpretations on the behavior. Anything from depression and sociopathic tendencies, but most of all, for attention.

So today, in my late thirties, I better understand the reasons behind the maladaptive behavior. The main reasons, for me, are guilt and to try and stop the feelings. There are some situations where I commit this heinous act for other reasons such as being challenged and sometimes attention.

For the guilt side of things, it doesn't take much to make me do it. It's not that I have to feel complete and utter shame to where I can no longer show my head in public. It could be the smallest amount of guilt, any guilt really. The only thing driven by the amount is how bad I hurt myself. Just some scratches or in situations like cheating on my partners, stiches and blood poisoning.

Nobody can stop me from feeling guilty either. No amount of kind words or "it's not your faults" can take it away. Granted, I may smile at those trying in the meantime but it stews and stews in me like a whirlpool. Just spinning and spinning until finally, sucked under in need of a way back to the surface.

There was only once where the guilt did not end in hurting myself. Once! I had cheated on my fiancé' while he was away AGAIN. Fortunately, my tattoo artist friend- the gentleman that covers the scars- got word of my indiscretion and that next morning, straight away. I had an 'S' tattooed into my chest in honor of my fiancé. I was fortunate enough to still hold the guilt but be able to act on it in a safe manner.

Then I bring you to the reason of "just needing to turn it off." This reason is a bit abstract because it could be a number of things I need to turn off. I might need to turn off the illusions, or the noise, or just zone everyone and everything around me out. This type of hurt gets it to stop. Sometimes.

The most prevalent thing I need to stop is needless fighting with my partners, and lately my fiancé. When I realize that the pushing and battering has gone too far (mainly from me and not him) I turn to the razors. I punish myself for letting it drag on too far and for turning him into the monster I see (don't worry, he doesn't actually become a monster although he does yell a lot and restrain me- it's just how I see him when I'm so angry that my head will throb and my ear drums will pound). I clench my teeth so badly sometimes that they will break and I will shake uncontrollably. I find the razors make these things stop. I find myself thinking they will fix everything. They never have and never will. But regardless, the thought is there at the time.

For the other reasons such as attention and being challenged. Those don't happen too often because fortunately

I am surrounded by many people that can "read" me and see when these situations might be occurring. THEY fix the situation, never me. Although I am slowly learning to ask for the help or attention I need.

Although for example sake (and yes, I've coined that very incorrect statement) I take you to the aforementioned night that had me put into therapy this most recent time. I had started a fight with Seth, accusing him of cheating as usual with no discernible proof. So, we got into it, the yelling and name calling, me chasing him around the apartment to yell and throw things. The usual. I had hurt myself with fortunately a very dull razor and then more arguing ensued between Seth and I, now on the topic of me hurting myself and how stupid it was. I had picked up a brand-new paring knife out of the silverware drawer. One thing led to another, and as he walked out on to the back porch for a cigarette I heard, "go ahead do it. I don't care." He challenged me.

I had hurt myself so badly it landed me in the back of a police car on the way to the hospital for stitches. There is nothing scarier than coming down from an episode with a kitchen full of EMTs, police officers and blood. I almost died that night but was lucky enough to end up with 12 stitches and much discomfort rather than a tomb stone. And this was just one of many nights like that.

Either reason for hurting myself has left my body with scars that will never heal, always be seen, and everywhere. My legs, my arms, my stomach, my chest and even my hands. Looking in the mirror every day causes me more shame than that which caused them to begin with. These scars will always be seen and judged. I will always be seen and judged.

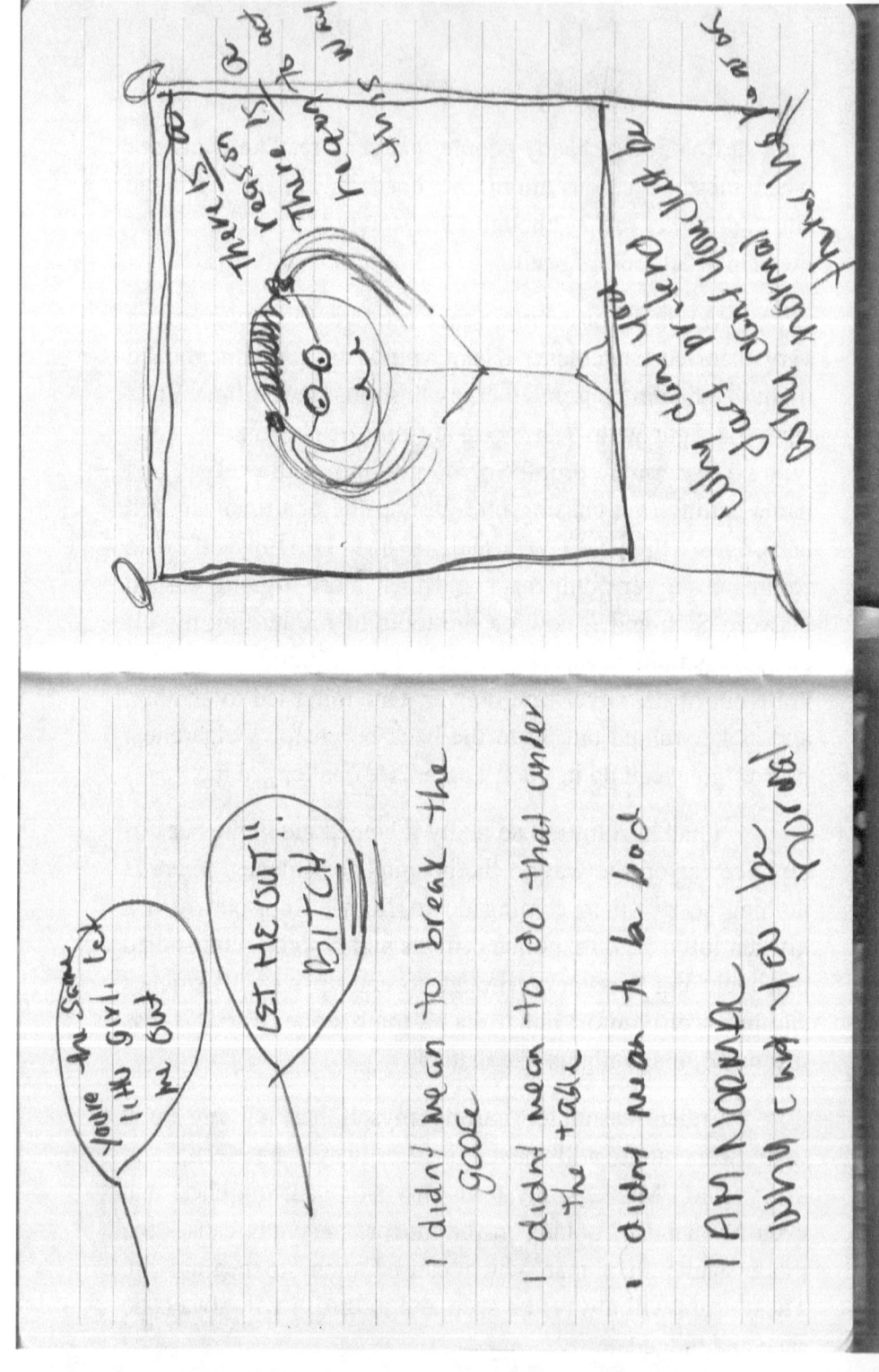

72

8/15

I see you looking into her face
and she is smiling at you - her smile
as you thrust into her

You put your dirty cock
into her. laugh at me

She laughs at me she
laughs at me

dirty cock
dirty cock
dirty cock

I want dirty
Was dirty
Dirty for
Cotton start
thank you
thank you
whatever you
like you

girl dirty
want want
want

"

Pain
Embrace because this is your life
Or does it mean breathing
And alive

The heartache you see is not me
I'm fierce
And something different
Than broken

Something more than broken
Great and strong
But dying
All the same

Butterflies fly
Infants coo
People laugh
But some ...

... some cower

"

IN THE END, CONCLUSION, FINAL WORDS OF WISDOM

In conclusion, my life is not terrible (in fact it is quite good) and I am typically the essence of 'sun shiny' but it requires a lot of strength and internal bullying to keep the days from beating me beyond control. I see everything. I notice the littlest of changes from the sound of my alarm clock to the look in my neighbor's eyes. If you can imagine, that makes life hard.

I will spend days arguing with myself and pacing holes in the floor because I am so bored and anxious that time stands still without a thing to do. I will spend other days so depressed that I must force myself to get dressed or eat. Other days I will be so manic that credit cards and car keys must be hid. I lose the ability to control my destiny, that's been taken away from me.

My doctor told me just the other day that my luck is running out and I am going to die. That was probably the hardest thing I have ever heard but it won't be true. I will prove her wrong because unlike most in my situation I am blessed to have such good friends, a fiancé that tries to take care of me, and an adopted family to call my own. Sadly, I have, at least once, done something terrible against most of those that have stuck around.. I never quite know why they stay. On the other hand, and this is what a lot of people in my situation, with my diagnosis, face. People leave, and they leave quickly and often. Some don't even stick around long enough to see the 'you' passed the scars.

But I lucked out. I have a best friend of almost 20 years that stuck by me even when I faltered and left her with a scar that she might never mend. Even when I've left her in the wake of all the self-punishments, anger, all the men and heartbreak. I can honestly say I couldn't live my life without her. If there was one thing (well two) that I could say to her it would be "I love you my dear friend and thank you."

I have my fiancé, Seth, that has faced aggression, accusations, sadness and blood. He has been my friend for a long time and in that time always kept me as safe as he could and always listened. He has stuck by me for three years of me telling him he's cheating on me with absolutely no proof and he still stays by my side, picks up the blood, and tries to convince me he's not cheating. He tries so hard to convince me that he let me put a tracker on his cell phone, calls me at every break and gave me all his passwords. What I would say to him and I feel I don't tell him this enough is "Thank you for what you do. Thank you for trying so hard and making me feel that I not only earned and deserve love, but I should demand it without cause because I am worth it."

To my father. I don't blame you for your part in my upbringing. I never did. You did the best you could with what you were given. And what you were given was a sick daughter who didn't know who she was, often where she was and what she was feeling. You never hit me, barely yelled at me but you were just hardly there and even when you were physically there you were hardly present. My statement to my father, "I love you dad and I'm ok."

AND NOW FOR THE SHORT STORIES- VERY SHORT IN FACT

I decided to include a couple of my short stories because they portray what a lot of people can't understand or don't want to see. They also portray things that I've wished for. An alter ego of sorts. Sometimes I could daydream up stories for hours about being something different. Someone different.

In my daydream I had strength and a normie wasn't the best thing to be. I'm slowly learning that broken makes me who I am. I may be judgmental if I didn't have my own scars, I may be mean if I didn't feel everything too much. Ernest Hemingway once said "We are all broken. That's how the light gets in."

,

I was born rich of two souls

some say I have not one.

One likes to bury the flesh and one likes to have fun

Take it from me

What I have to give

One face, two face

Nothing in place

One soul or two

Ones got trouble up his sleeve

The other didn't pull through.

They Call Me Tiff. Chapter I

They call me Tiff- and this my story.

My village does not take well to the strange and unusual folk… so they built a house made of stone and steel. This house has no windows, no flowers greeting the strongly barricaded door, and barely a light. Hidden away from the remaining beauty of the village where it can be ignored and forgotten. This house…. this is where I live.

My parents sent me to live here with the other misunderstood when I was just a young girl of barely six years on this Earth. They would not admit the faceless figure in my slumber could be a real- living and breathing- being. This masked person I looked to every night was out there and our souls were calling to each other but my parents denied the possibility… instead they feared me abnormal and locked me away. I feel as though, I may have been crazy, but I feel much more strongly that my parents were hiding something much different than fear of their progeny darkening their name. I feel as though they knew such a veiled being would preoccupy my dreams… but why?

It was a day- like any other day. There was a warm wind breezing through the dense trees and quite a few birds and insects coloring our world with various buzzes and chirps. All the strange folk were spending their afternoon enjoying the slivers of sunlight as they beamed through the tiny portholes and lit up the great room. I was laying against the East wall drawing numbers in the carpet- pretending as though it was a chalkboard and I was teaching a class of young ones not yet tainted by the throws of the village into assuming us misunderstood folk belong outside of society.

These young minds had much to learn so it was good that I had several hours to spare before dinner.

A startling static sang from the television and the chirps and buzzes stopped. In a gasp some of the others and I ran to the portholes in time to see that the trees had also stopped moving- the world had stopped. Several of us panicked, some ran in circles, some hid under chairs warning the rest of us of doomsday. All the gasping and cries stopped when a shadowy figure appeared towards the middle of the great room. It was more solid than a shadowy figure would be expected to be but not quite there. All the others were frozen in either fear or wonder- it was so hard to tell with them sometimes.

The smart half of me knew that I should just ignore the figure or fear it- but not get closer. The smarter half was beaten as I inched my way to the shadowy figure. I was in awe at how lifeless a shadow is but how full of life this creature seemed. I continued to creep closer and closer and suddenly the shadowy figure turned to face me. I could clearly see now, a man behind the shadow. He was still veiled and diverse, but a man all the same. "Ah…. There you are", he said, "it won't be long now that I've found you".

"Who are you?" I replied, "how are you doing this?"

"You don't remember do you? Anything at all?"

"Who are you? How do you know me?" I asked again.

"Two lay as one then one lay alone. You are not who you think little Veritas."

    Just as quickly as he came, the shadowed man disappeared. I wondered to myself who he was and more importantly what he meant. "Two lay as one then one lay alone" could mean many a thing- or not a thing at all. I remembered learning about riddles during one of the Sunday book ventures before I was sent to live here. That sounded like a riddle, like any other. I thought I was smarter than to be duped by a shadowed man randomly appearing in our great room… but he knew me. How did he know me? I've known nothing more than the people here and those living lives as free-men down in the village. I would remember that voice… but I do remember that voice. Nobody I have met has that voice!

    Things were becoming far too complicated and clouded so I welcomed and found myself thankful for the dinner that was being wheeled into the hallway on its way to the dining room. A welcome sight. We all started to head out of the great room- some shoving involved- towards the dining room. I customarily fell behind the crowd to make it less the ordeal as it should be. There was always plenty of seating and plenty to eat that there was no need to push myself through the crowd as others had grown accustomed. On my way to the hall, I heard an odd chirp from the far side of the wall. It was not a sickly or angered chirp, but odd all the same. I made my way to the far porthole to see if I can spot the creature that made such a chirp only to find a single bee rested on the outside landing of the stone frame. Not hurt, not flying, just sitting there. "What an odd thing to see," I thought to myself. The closer I got, the bee still stayed without an attempt to fear or question my intent.

"Tiff- are you coming to dinner? You need to eat." One of the house maids called after me.

I left the lonely bee in peace and made my way to the dining room. The chairs were filled and the table was piled. The other misunderstood had wasted no time filling their plates- and mouths- some causing disorder by stealing from other's plates and reaching for their glasses. I sat at the far end of the table and had all intentions to start to my meal but I just could not stop thinking about the shadowed man and now that lonely bee without reason to be where either of them were supposed to be.

"Housemother?" I asked aloud. "What is a vare- i- toss?"

"Oh dear Tiff- wherever did you hear that?" Housemother replied.

"I heard it somewhere quite recently and I believe I have heard it in the lesson books before but cannot place it."

"Well... Veritas is the goddess of truth. She would let others see the unhidden around them, the truth in things. She could let others see the beaten wife, the sad child. But you need not worry Tiff as she hid herself away in a well so deep that others could never find her. And if they could not find her she could not make them see. "

"But housemother" I replied, "why would we want her to be hidden so deep in a well that she could not make others see the truth in things?"

Housemother thought a good many seconds for her best response to speedily end this conversation. She finally responded, "Well... sometimes folks are not prepared for what's really in front of them. Sometimes it's easier that way, sometimes the truth can be painful and scary. Now please, go ahead and eat your supper before it gets cold so we can all wash up for bed."

I did as housemother had requested and picked at the food on my plate until I appropriately ate enough to appease the others. As the plates were being cleared, we all made our way to the upstairs dorms. The top floor was separated into two sections, both sharing a series of bathrooms. Men were on the right and women on the left. I snuck into one of the bathrooms with a couple of the other girls to brush my teeth and wash my face before bed. The two girls were speaking of the shadowed man as if he was any other man that had just come for a visit from outside the village- as people from the village rarely visited us misunderstood behind the stone walls. "He was so dreamy," one of the girls said in response to the second girl asking her opinion. Then as if they were aware of one another's thoughts, they both turned to me to question how I had known him. "But I do not know him," I responded. When both the catty dorm mates said in harmony, "He certainly knows you." I would have otherwise been annoyed at their frankness but they were entirely accurate- he does know me.

I finished up in the bathroom as quickly as I could, put my towel on the rack to dry for morning, and hurried to bed. The dorm beds were racked side by side three by six. Fortunately, the two catty girls laid bunk on the far side of the dorm, closest to the windows. I was hoping for a good solid sleep tonight since my last few had been anything but. Unexpectedly, as if someone had struck me, I heard a voice.

"Think Tiffany, think. Remember. I need you to see now little Veritas. I need you to see the masks, the flowers, and the forever. Wake up little Veritas. It's your time now"

I shuddered awake from the voice, as if an alarm had triggered inside me. Who is this man? Why do I not know of which he speaks? I decided, since I would not actually be able to fall back to sleep, to read a little bit by what little moonlight buffed through the far window- next to the catty girls. Fortunately, they were deep in slumber, no doubt dreaming of ponies and rainbows. Morning would come soon enough, followed by breakfast, and then more time spent in the great room. The story I was engulfing myself in, unfortunately, was not very entertaining. At least not entertaining enough to free my mind from the shadowed man and the voices I've heard since.

Now trying very little to pay attention to my otherwise inviting book, I peered out the window into the beautifully manicured lawn below. Then I noticed him… the shadowed man… was once again so close. It was if he was waiting for me out past the front- strongly barricaded door- to run to him. Even if I could get past housemother's room and the door blockades- what would I say? How would I refer to the mere fact that he is a shadow? Am I crazy? How am I even considering this?

As quick as the thought to run had come, my muscles chose to decide for me. I turned and ran from the room, no thought of the interruptions I may be causing the others' sleep. I hung to the doorframe as I peered towards housemother's room and quietly crept towards the stairwell, avoiding any creaks possible as not to alert anyone of my treachery. I swiftly tiptoed down the stairs towards the front door- the only obstacle between me and the shadowed man. As I stood, overwhelmed by the complication now directly in front of me, the comforting noises invariably resting inside my mind settled. I felt very uneasy at the sudden silence- this was not normal. Was I having a stroke? Did all that sneaking, and worry give me a stroke?

Then unpredictably, I heard a single voice where all my friendly noise had once premiered. "Veritas", it called out to me, "Tiff…."

"You know how to open the door… you know Tiff."

"But <u>how</u>?" I quietly whispered in response without knowing if this was the stroke or if I could truly be heard.

"The door is holding you in by nothing more than magic Tiff. Those needing to be behind those walls are locked away because they truly need to be behind those walls. Their minds aren't right, they have a sickness. The door- the obstacle in front of you- is spelled to hold the sick and their elected wardens in. Those who are not sick can just open the door as if no lock- no magic exists- to keep it shut."

"If that is true... then I am trapped as well. I am stuck behind these walls because my mind isn't right... my mind is sick." Tears started to well in my eyes as I began to remember the look on my mother's face when she recognized that I was one of the misunderstood. I started to remember the day that they dropped me here and never looked back at me as they took the carriage back through the long drive towards the village.

"Open.... The ..... Door ....Veritas. Just turn the handle. <u>Now</u>!"

"I <u>can't</u>," I exclaimed in not the intended whisper as I turned to run back up the stairs and pretend to slumber before any punishment befell me. I heard no response- I was relieved and very saddened all at once.

I crept past housemother's room once again and fell to the nearest bunk I could find. Wrapped in my blankets-safe and unseen. I laid awake for a while, wondering about what had just transpired, wondering about the shadowed man, until I relaxed enough to close my eyes until morning. A good six hours had passed before I was woken by the common chirps and buzzes that mark the daylight hours. There were no dreams that I could recall and no whispers in my sleep. It was a restful sleep- a good sleep.

I started to gather my clothes and wash things to clean up before breakfast when out of the blue I looked up from my bedside table and one of the younger girls was standing in front me of me in wonder and shouted at me as if the sounds were so loud in the room that no one around could hear. "I had the strangest dream!" she yelled. It seemed I would not be getting to the washroom or breakfast anytime soon. I offered the girl a spot at the end of the bunk so she could tell me what was apparently a very important dream.

She started on… "I think I was in a park by one of those merry-go-rounds and there were two kids coloring on one of those benches. A boy and a girl? Yep- a boy and a girl. They were my age! The boy was kind of cute but don't tell housemother that. I could hear them talking but I wasn't close so they must have talked real loud- like. The boy was asking the girl why she wouldn't draw him a picture so he can hang it with his knight collector cards. He seemed very sad…. I would draw him a picture. The girl said that she only draws things that are going to happen or have happened that others can't see- or they don't see... I don't remember her exact words. And then the boy asked her if she won't draw him a picture how come she'll never fold him a paper rose. Then it got kind of sad... the girl told the boy that she

86

promised him she would fold him a paper rose before he went away so she won't make him one or else he'll leave."

As the little girl went on I could almost picture the park in my head. I could almost picture this boy. Where had I seen a park like that before? I don't remember ever going to a park when I was down in the village with my parents. I would love to have sat in a park on a nice warm day and colored but mother and father never let me color. All the pencils and paints were locked up in our house- they were very strict on things I couldn't do or play with. "You're not listening," the girl called out as she continued with her story.

"The boy asked to see what she had drawn and before she could tuck it away with the others he grabbed it out of her hand. I could not see what it was but it made the boy very angry and he started to yell at the girl... then he started to cry."

As if some flash had hit me I quickly snapped at the girl "What did he yell?" "Geez", the girl replied as she continued her story. "The boy started yelling about how she can't let her parents do something. Something about a doctor and what the doctor can do to him. As the boy started yelling louder and louder all the nearby faces turned to look. An older man with the meanest face rushed towards the two and started pulling the girl's arm. I think he was hurting her and she kept dragging her shoes into the ground- you know by the heel. The boy was trying to push the man but he just didn't seem large enough. Then finally right before I woke up the boy yelled louder than he had yet... and I can't really remember now what he said but it was something about they can never make her forget him because she is a Vare-toes?"

"Veritas?", I replied, probably much more of a shout than intended. "That's it- that's the word", she excitedly responded. "Can I go to breakfast now?" she asked. I responded with a polite thank you and a nod and before I could look towards the girl the little girl had flown past headed to the dining hall. I should have been heading there myself but I couldn't wrap my mind around the shadowed man and <u>now</u> the little girl's dream referring to another as the same thing- Veritas- seer of truth as housemother explained. "How could this all be? This is all so crazy." I thought to myself. I must try and get these things out of my head. Mother and father always told me trying to look too much into things would lead to trouble or sadness. Both of which us misunderstood should avoid given our current living arrangements.

I decided to smarten up and try and hold the thoughts and go about my day. I grabbed my washcloth and toothbrush and headed towards the bathroom. The day seemed like any other. I could hear clanging and commotion down the stairs towards the dining room and saw the maids scampering about. Fortunately everyone had already made use of the washrooms so I had no line or crowd to wade through. I washed up, brushed my teeth and then hurried back to the dorm to drop my things off and throw on some shoes. So far the morning is turning out uneventful- a welcome juncture.

Breakfast too was uneventful besides getting scolded for being late. Housemother always appreciates punctuality but fortunately her scolding is nothing more than a firm "Tiff" and a raised eyebrow. I ate my breakfast, drank my juice and hurried over to the great room to get the best seat for the morning announcements. This morning however, the static was not playing over the radio, instead a strange man- I would assume from the village was standing in the front of the room with a series of papers in his hand.

"Are we all here?" he said signaling housemother.

She looked around the room before responding, "Yes, sir everyone seems accounted for."

"Good," he said in response. "We can continue." He took a brief second looking around the room, seemingly avoided eye contact with any of us as the villagers often did. "Unfortunately this morning's typical radio announcement is canceled due to some incidents down in the village. These incidents are dreadful and confusing but rest assured the lawmen are doing everything in their power to find more answers and stop this travesty from continuing."

The room started to get very rowdy before the stranger could continue. He beckoned to housemother for a little assistance in quieting the commotion. Within a few minutes, the room was quieted again and the man continued speaking.

"We are not sure how this has happened or who is involved but several villagers seemed to have gone missing throughout the night. The only clues we are finding is a single rose folded from paper left outside their door. Some of the people that have gone have relatives right in this room which is why I am here. I will list the names without question than be on my way." I could feel the panic fill the room and some of the misunderstood were already starting to shake before the unfriendly strange man began to list off names. "I'd appreciate if you let me get through the lists without any outburst and then I will hand it over to your housemother." He said as once again beckoning to housemother.

"We will do just that sir," she said as she nodded her head towards each row of us.

"Franklin and Georgiana Waldorf- Jeffrey and Yana Mistole- Oliver and Andrea Joyce- Michael and Evelyn Geofries- and finally Icabod and Henrietta Luttel"

Several of the misunderstood started to wale as the names were called. Some started sobbing uncontrollably and then a couple of the others began to smile and laugh. Unfortunately, I do not know many of my dorm mates' families but I'm assuming that by the reactions they were somewhere in that list. I looked up for comfort from anyone apart from the waling only to see housemother- as promised- rushing the stranger to the front door; Presumably to ride away in his fancy carriage.

"Tiffany Luttle," housemother called as she returned from the front door, barging her way back into the great room, "Tiff? ... Oh there you are! Come with me". Without hesitation I jumped up and hurriedly followed housemother into the hall. I gave her a few seconds to catch her breath but was overcome with anticipation on what further news comes- as if the first bit didn't do me in enough for one day.

"Tiff. The gentleman that was just here with the news told me that the clue left behind from your parents' home was a little more than the others," housemother said as she held a piece of paper in her hand. "Here", she continued, "I have not read it yet. I feel it is only right that you read first." I carefully unfolded the rose that was left behind from the people that took my parents. It was a different rose from the others with much writing on all sides. A very small, neat script made it easy to tell it was not left on a whim. It's as if it was prewritten.

The note seemed to be mostly nonsensical but there were some parts that caught my attention. The note went on to say how those that were taken were because they offered no benefit to the village and surrounding towns. Not only that but it continued to portray how they were less than a benefit to their children and those they've left behind. How every man and woman taken harmed their own families in one way or another. My parents, worst of all. It carried on about how my parents knew I was special and that I had belonged somewhere different and instead they cast me out as one of the misunderstood where I'd be raised by a housemother and nurses. Never knowing the true depth I had or my real belonging. The final passage written should have made no sense but I couldn't stop reading over and over. It read "Your legs have walked before; your sharp tongue has caused trouble before; your lips have lain on mine before; your legs have trembled for me before; you are alive again- for me- as I you. Veritas. Remember."

As I looked up from the note both sorrowful and confused I noticed housemother with an interested glow about her. She was a kind lady but very stern and typically didn't take to her housemates seemingly as dazed as I must have been- but she was accepting it aside her curiosity. "Housemother", I asked, "does this make sense to you? It seems as though it's familiar but I have never laid eyes on such a verse." Without even a glance at the note- that which she had never seen, housemother replied, "Sweetheart... it's time to go. You must remember. That note is a reminder. A reminder that you, my dear, have never belonged behind these walls. I'm growing old and tired and cannot keep watch any longer. He has come for you at just the right time. It's up to you now." Then housemother turned away and slunk up the stairs towards her room. I was even more confused- there were so many unanswered questions. Did housemother know the shadowed man that have been haunting us or did she know what any of this meant. Oh how I wish she would have told me what any of this meant should she know.

Gripping the note tightly as if it were the last testament of a dying race, I decided after all the commotion that now would be a good time for a short afternoon nap. I headed upstairs without a peep around the room to see if others had paid mind of the commotion between housemother and me. I decided to lay rest on one of the far bunks so I could feel the afternoon glow of the sun that shined perfectly through the back windows. Surprisingly enough, sleep came quick. Perhaps it was because of the calmness in housemother's voice when she told me I did not belong here or maybe the stress of the whole morning ordeal and the sorrow for the disappearance of my parents. I had almost forgotten about them. Not surprisingly, the dreams also came quick.

I was standing outside of what seemed to be an old formation of boulders and Earth. I could feel the fresh breeze as it rustled my hair just enough to tickle my cheeks. I looked behind me as I recognized rusting through branches some distance away and then I saw him coming up over the hill. He so closely resembled the shadowed man without the hidden grace. He was striking. He had such strong features and as he got closer, I could gaze upon the most beautiful eyes this world had ever seen. He stood before me with a sharp smile as if he had just cracked the most vulgar joke. Before I had chance to mutter a sound, he reached his arm behind me and pulled me closer. With a firm yet such graceful manner he placed his lips on mine. I could feel my heart racing and my body temp rising as he tentatively traced his tongue against my bottom lip. He held firmer as he lowered me onto the dew-soaked Earth and gently kneeled over me leaning down between glances to kiss me yet again. Each kiss growing more and more intense until finally he leaned backwards one more time and drew his hand closer to my body and...

"Tiff- <u>wake up</u>" housemother was shouting from the dorm door. "You are causing a ruckus downstairs. What were you dreaming?" I shot up out of bed and ran to the stairs. All around the ground floor were the misunderstood running around dancing and kissing and <u>touching</u> each other. I was so confused and looked to housemother for some guidance. "Tiff- calm down and think about something other than the feelings in your dream." As I started to cycle through thoughts less provoking, things like puppies and dinner with family and doing chores that housemother often required of us I could hear the commotion also quieting downstairs. This was all so confusing- the dream that felt like I had been there before and done just that with that unbelievable man before and now this... housemother treating the problem with the rest of the housemates as if it was something I alone caused.

"Housemother, I do not understand. What you meant, what the note meant, how my dream.... How my dream could do that." As if she refused to give explanation or if she had not even listened to my sorrowful inquiry housemother turned towards the stairs and made her way down to the front door. "Come," she called, "come here Tiff." I descended the stairs as housemother had instructed still hoping she may shed some kind of enlightenment.

"Open the door, "she instructed further. The same as I had argued with the shadowed man I responded, "But housemother, it's spelled." She replied, "Only against the sick Tiff. Not those like me and certainly not those like you. Just try it Tiff. It won't hurt." Hesitantly I reached for the doorknob and started to turn. Half expecting to be shocked or burned I cringed away as I pulled the door towards me. It opened, the door knob turned and the heavily barricaded door opened for me. I turned to housemother hoping for some guidance on the next steps or a reminder of what being outside these walls were like. As if she understood the fear that must be quite visible in my appearance she calmly instructed, "You go out this door and you start walking towards the tree line across the yard. He will come to you, and you will remember my perfect Tiff. The world's perfect Veritas." And she gestured me out the door without another word and I could hear the strong door latch behind me.

In front of me stood the rest of the world that was hidden behind the stone walls. There was more intrigue and desire ahead of me than there was confusion and fright. What was to become of me? Where was I to go from here? I made my way across the yard to the tree line as housemother had instructed and there he was- in the clearing of the sunlight glow. The shadowed man. My shadowed man.

"There you are Veritas. This time took much longer than that others. I thought you'd never see."

... to be continued

Untitled. Story !

Amid a little village there was a great mansion. The mansion belonged to the most famed local merchant and his daughter Rea. The merchant was tyrannical when he ran his household and insisted, since his daughter had become of marrying age, that she was to settle only for one of the more royal of the local boys her age. The merchant would not have Rea sully the family name by falling for some local riff-raff as she had done in the past. Well as the stories go, only the fairest surprising locals will win her heart.

One day when the sun was shining exceptionally bright, Rea decided to walk to the market for an icy dream. Icy dreams were fantastic concoctions with frozen bananas and blueberry juice. On the way to the market Rea noticed a young man, a bit older than she was but not by much.

The man she spotted was covered in soot and atop a ladder cleaning the gutters for the local inn. As she walked past the gentlemen he glanced down and noticed her delightful stare.

"Who is that man?" Rea though to herself. "There's something about him I just can't seem to place". You see the man was common, no discernible features aside from a set of beautiful slate-blue eyes. But ordinary all the same. Not like the handsome boys her father insisted on her settling with. Plain and ordinary- but there was something.

As he glanced down at Rea she turned away in embarrassment, he gathered a half-smile and watched as her rosy cheeks grew rosier. "She's not like the other girls" he thought to himself. Turned from her rosy cheeks and went back to the gutter work ahead of him.

Rea was still in awe as she made her way past the market stalls. "What was so special about that man?" She just couldn't place it. Regardless, she went on to the market stall where she would find her "Icy Dream". The line was quite long as expected given the state of the heat that day. But it would be well worth the wait.

Suddenly she found herself compelled towards the road where nothing more than a crowd had just gathered. She saw him again. The dirt on his jeans reached all the way to his boots and eventually the ground. His cheeks were brushed with soot and his lips chapped in the sun. He had been looking down at the ground at a rock he had been kicking while waiting for the market stall to free of its long line of people when he must have felt the same compulsion to look up. He caught Rea once more with a glimmering look in her eye as she stared.

When unexpectedly he started to make his way over to the "Icy Dream" stall where Rea stood waiting. She noticed him walking in her direction and thought to herself, "oh goodness. I hope he's not after me. Father wouldn't have it and I don't feel the need of associating with such a man just because there's something about him I can't place". Well, not long after she did realize he was after her attention. Although she couldn't possibly associate with such a man she was intrigued as to her recent infatuation with him.

"My name's Joseph", the man said while reaching out his hand to Rea. Rea could not possibly allow the man to grab her hand. He was a stranger with soot from head to toe and she was a lady who listened to her father's wishes. But whatever it was, she found the need to touch the man. She wanted to jump into his arms and have him whisk her away. "But I couldn't possibly", she thought to herself.

Instead she reached out and allowed this Joseph to grab her hand after all. He placed her hand in his ever so gently- not to move it past the length of her fingers. "He has the most ferocious look but the gentlest grasp" she thought to herself. How could such a man not have caught my eye before. The more she looked up at him his darkened sooty features became almost a sense of art. An unfounded beauty. And his eyes, his eyes told stories while looking so cold at the same time. She still cannot figure what is so special about Joseph other than being a stranger with beautiful eyes and the most carnal grasp.

"Hello Joseph" she exclaimed, "I am Rea".

"The merchant's daughter", Joseph replied. "I imagine your father would not be too keen on you conversing with the likes of me".

Rea had no response, but he was correct in his assumption of what her father would deem appropriate. Joseph would certainly not fall in the very small bucket her father deemed worthy of his lovely daughter.

Joseph saw that Rea had no response for his forthcoming remark about her father's disapproval so to save her the agony of trying to muster a response, he continued the conversation.

"Rea," he said, "come take a walk with me, won't you?"

Against her better judgement Rea agreed and stepped out of line at the market stall and paid no mind to the stares surrounding her. Her father would certainly be told about this and she would surely hear it when she returned home. She couldn't stay away, she must find out what Joseph has to offer. He seemingly whispered such a glimmer of light through what seemed to be permanent soot on his face and clothes. As she walked away with this stranger, this mess, this amazing creature a few gasps rose from the line around them. "Now father will certainly hear," she thought to herself.

The two of them walked hand in hand through the village. Rea paid no mind to the gasps and stares. She just looked up at Joseph and she felt the smallest tickle in her chest. Something she had never felt before. She did not know if he was bad- or good. Whether he had ill intentions- or harmless ones. All she knew was that she felt something and WAS something. They said no words, but words were not needed. He grasped her hand tighter and tighter as they walked, and she could feel his intentions. As suspected, they were pure but different. Like him.

Joseph continued down the road and she knew where he was taking her once again, without words. They had come to a clearing and through the clearing was the smallest stream. This path was off limits because of the river's habitual offenses towards the safety of the villagers. She did not care. She had this vigilant feeling that he would protect her should something happen.

They finally reached the end of the clearing and the bridge overlooking the river. The bridge was once used to transport heavy metals from the refining factory to the neighboring towns for sales. It had not seen horses or buggies in quite some time. The pressed gravel was dented with years of rain and the side mound had started to wash away.

Joseph twirled Rea around to seat her on the cleanest part of the once beautiful stone benches and knelt in front of her. "Why would you not have a seat", Rea asked. "Because conversing with such a beautiful lady deems it necessary to sit afront not beside"

"Rea, you must understand something," Joseph began to explain. "I am not like all the other villagers. Neither the ones in fancy garb or those covered in grime as I am."

"What is it?" Rea exclaimed.

"I was born different my beautiful Rea. Please you must try and keep an open mind".

Rea jumped up for Joseph to follow-suit. She wanted nothing more than to jump in his arms. She didn't care what was different about him, just that it was. She tired of the boring and same and Joseph was right, He was different.

But as Rea jumped up preparing to dive into Josephs arms, she saw something. There was the faintest shade beside her that moved as she moved.

"Is that a shadow?" she questioned.

"Yes, sweet Rea" Joseph replied. "That's what I was trying to tell you"

For you see, the villagers all lost their shadows long ago when they became like everyone else. Only happiness was allowed and deem fit for the village and any outliers must be sent away or domesticated.

"Joseph," Rea asked, "you are my shadow?"

"No. My beautiful Rea. I am not your shadow"

"Then you gave me my shadow back," Rea exclaimed in excitement. "You have given me back myself. No more hiding Joseph for you have given me my shadow back!"

"No." Joseph replied again. "I did not give you your shadow either. You have been there all along, through the good days and the hidden ones. That's what I was trying to tell you. There's something different about me. My soul wants to see the truth in things, in people. I did not give you your shadow, I simply move the darkness out of the way so your shadow can return."

"Can the others get their shadows back as well", Rea questioned. "Can you move the darkness for them too?"

"Unfortunately, not beautiful Rea," Joseph explained, "for you see not everyone is ready to step out of the darkness. Your light still had glimmer through all of it you still had hope. And not hope for yourself but hope for all the other villagers as well. Hope for life."

"But if I return with my shadow, I shall be judged for being different and send from the village"

"Show them who you are Rea. Show them that being different is not bad. Show them shadows mean something. You see shadows are not good or bad, they do not scar with their owners, but they do laugh with them."

Rea and Joseph returned to the village and as Rea expected to be rejected it was not the response she received. The other villagers flocked to Rea and wanted to know how she was suddenly so different than everyone. The children laughed and jumped upon Rea's shadow as if it was a great big puddle after a silent rain.

Rea realized that sometimes you can be different, and people would surprise you in many ways. She kept her shadow for a long time and her and Joseph along with her shadow landed in a big house with a big bright lawn where she would run back and forth all the while her shadow chasing her.

07/12

Why do you keep feeding
the episodes? you are
such a hateful PRICK

you have no idea what
you even do wrong

Stop laughing
Stop laughing
Stop laughing
Stop laughing loudly

Cushing

07/08

he must have hated

Such a long time without

her but no worries there
Swamp stank - He made
Sure to save himself up

Just for you !?!

05/29

He denies or doesn't do how
he changes from the man!
love - the man only that place 2d5

to what makes me feel hated
and betrayed and unloved.
The thing that makes me
walk on eggshells - the thing
that makes me hate him.
Fuckins piece of shit

I watch it every day.
You're fun, you're crazy
You're happy and ok
Sam as its about time

to see me

Hate yourself
Fake it fake
Hate yourself
Hate

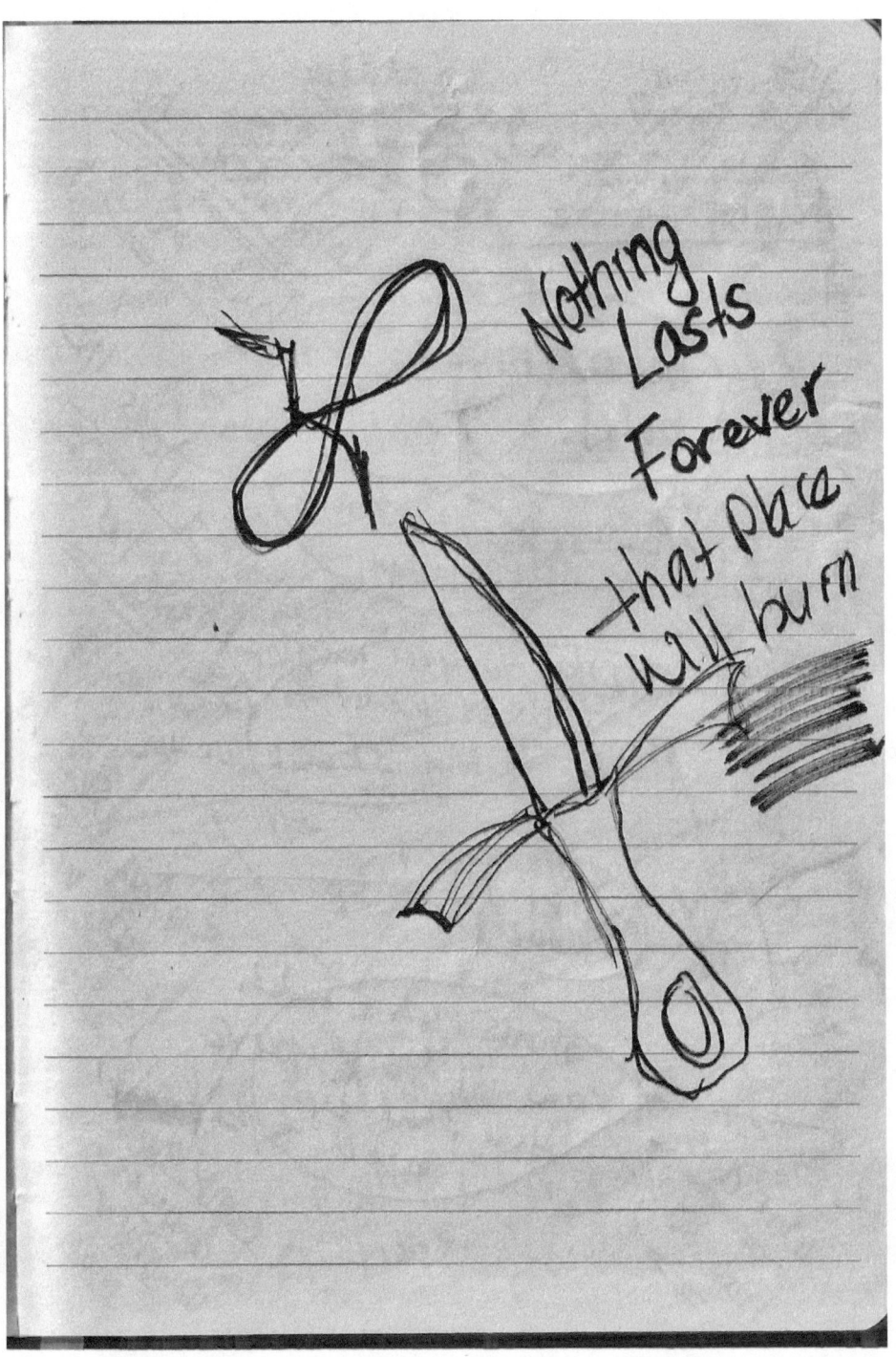

What will I drink
tomorrow?
Run = he cloated
vodka = he cloated

www.ingramcontent.com/pod-product-compliance
Lightning Source LLC
Chambersburg PA
CBHW020545220526
45463CB00006B/2197

* 9 7 8 1 7 9 7 9 3 7 3 6 6 *